LIFELONG

Stronger, Faster, Leaner, Smarter, Sexier—At Any Age

Jerry Mixon, MD

The information in this book has been carefully researched, and all efforts have been made to ensure accuracy. The author and publisher assume no responsibility for any injuries suffered or damages or losses incurred during or because of following the program in this book. Consult with your physician or qualified medical professional before beginning this or any health program. The information and advice presented in this book are not meant to substitute for the advice of your family's physician or other trained healthcare professionals. You are advised to consult with healthcare professionals about all matters pertaining to your health and well-being.

Copyright © 2023 by Jerry Mixon

All rights reserved.

Published in the United States by Patuxent River Press

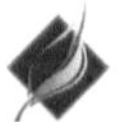

Library of Congress Cataloguing in Publication has been applied for.

Paperback ISBN: 979-8-9887421-1-1
Hardcover ISBN: 979-8-9887421-0-4
Ebook ISBN: 979-8-9887421-2-8

Printed in the United States of America
First Edition

For the millions of people who are suffering unnecessary disability and dying needlessly young. May this book be your first step toward a long and joyous life.

Contents

Introduction

Feel Younger/Live Better

This book is about how to live a *longer*, fuller, and more joyful life. It will show you how to reduce your risk of dementia, stroke, heart attack, diabetes, degenerative arthritis, and cancer. Equally important, it will tell you how you can have more sensual pleasures and passion in your life. Yes, Eros is a part of that, but when I say *passion*, I mean more than sex. I want you to increase your joy and enthusiasm in every aspect of your life. I suspect you have seen small children running for the sheer fun of it. You have heard them happily screaming and shouting over nothing more than jumping in puddles after a rainstorm. That childish passion for life is what too many adults have lost.

The reality is that it is hard to be that kid when your back aches, your hips or knees protest every step, or you just feel tired and gloomy. Add in your worries about politics, social changes, family issues, career, or retirement and it's no wonder it's difficult to be enthusiastic about life.

I've been a doctor since 1976 and I've learned that the truth about health, disease, and longevity—life and death issues—cannot be sugarcoated. The truth can be communicated with care and kindness, but the message has to be said boldly so it is fully understood. When I was younger, people weren't even told they had cancer for fear of "upsetting" them. They died in pain, confused, and often unable to get their affairs in order.

For that reason, this book uses a word that has become almost forbidden in polite society. Bear with me for a moment: The word is *fat*. When I use this word, I am absolutely *not* fat-shaming anyone. One of the critical truths we need to address is that *fat is not a person* or a moral state of being. When I say or write *fat*, I am referring to it as a tissue, just like skin and muscle are tissues. Fat is a part of us; it is *not* us. Fat is unique in that it functions as though it were a gland and produces more than 80 different peptides, hormones, cytokines, and immune factors that have a massive impact on our health and, critically, on our mood. Most people do not realize that fat triggers depression and fatigue in addition to that dangerous list of maladies I listed in the second sentence of this book.

We need to face the truth; we have an enormous health problem in this country. Our life spans are declining. In 1900, life expectancy was 47 years. In 2019, it was 79. By 2021, it dropped to 76.4. This isn't just due to COVID or drug overdoses. It's also due to our poor health.

According to the National Institutes of Health, 75 percent of Americans over 50 are overweight or obese. In 1932, diabetes was found in one in every 147 people. The Centers for Disease Control currently says that one in *three* Americans will be diabetic at some point in their lives, because most are overweight to obese. For a doctor who cares about people, this is *terrifying*.

Is there something in human physiology that's changed in the last 90 years? *Nope*. What's changed is our diet and our lifestyle. Countless studies and statistics have shown that we could cut diabetes by 80 percent; dementia, heart disease, high blood pressure, kidney failure, and degenerative arthritis by 50 percent; and cancer by 20 percent . . . *if* we change how and what we eat. We could likely achieve the longevity we're longing for. All it takes is getting lean.

Now, you might be thinking, *That's a pretty dramatic statement*. But let me explain something to you about Mother Nature. She's no benign, benevolent earth mother. She's a mean, hard, selfish so-and-so who only cares about one thing, and it sure isn't you. She only cares about the survival of the species.

That's why human beings become weak, slow, fat, dumb, and sexless as we age. If it makes you feel any better, this isn't a recent phenomenon.

If you look at paintings of wealthy, middle-aged Europeans during the Renaissance, many of them were thick and overweight. But they weren't on our modern diet, with depleted soil and chemicals in their food. So something has been going on for centuries that made humans gain weight and lose muscle as they got older.

All due to Mother Nature, who decided humans need to have a sell-by date. She made us most fertile in our teen years, so we'd have our kids young and stay strong and durable until our children could have children. Once that happens, we're kaput from a biological standpoint; as soon as we die, resources are saved for the next generation. By our mid-30s, things start falling apart *because they're supposed to*. You're supposed to get weak, slow, fat, dumb, sexless . . . and dead!

Our hormones, the tools our bodies use to make us lean, fit, and strong, decline because Mother Nature pulls the plug on them. As our bodies are deprived of these tools that are necessary to grow strong, lean tissue, we become softer, rounder, and broader. If your body can no longer make muscles, bones, ligaments, tendons, and sinews, it will make fat tissue instead.

So stop blaming yourself if you feel crummy when you look in the mirror every morning and wonder why you can't lose the weight you know you need and want to lose. People's health and obesity problems are *not* just due to lifestyle or lack of willpower or the kind of moral failure fat-shamers like to spout. (Sometimes I think that Mother Nature has teamed up with food companies who know exactly how to tempt consumers with piles of tasty junk food by the checkout lines in the supermarkets.) Survival traits that kept our cave-dwelling ancestors alive are what's killing us now. Most of us don't realize *that losing weight is an inherently unnatural act*, so we need to use every trick we can to fool our minds and bodies.

That's where this book will help you. My goal is to incentivize, educate, and inspire you. If I can do it, so can you.

At the age of 50, I was Fat Jerry. I was round, soft, and depressed. I was damn near sexless. I had the hormone balance and lifestyle of a typical middle-aged, workaholic male. For the last 26 years, however, I've carried the hormone balance of a 25-year-old man, which gives me incredible metabolic advantages. Now, when I eat sensibly, I lose fat tissue. If I exercise, I make muscle. I'm doing everything I can to work my way around Mother Nature's plan that wants me to be a chubby, die tomorrow, and stop consuming resources that younger generations need.

If you want to live a long, robust, happy life, you cannot let that archaic caveman physiology have its way. I know what's it's doing to us and I know how to fix it. You just have to get off your butt and do it.

The Difference Between Health Span and Life Span

For most of human history, we stayed young and vigorous until dying before the age of 40 or so. Regular plagues swept through small villages and larger cities, putting all citizens at risk. Even centuries later, infant and child mortality rates were devastating. According to the CDC, in 1900, 30 percent of all American deaths were children younger than five. One hundred years later, that death rate was just 1.4 percent. In other words, until very recently, health span and life span were closely connected. Once you became sick, you quickly went downhill and died.

That's why, when Social Security was launched in the 1930s, 65 was set as the age when people could collect the money they had been paying into the system. The reason was simple: The average American life span was 47, so only about 5 or 6 percent of the American population was ever going to live long enough to get a payout. Those lucky seniors had longevity.

Here's the rub: Modern medicine has allowed us to extend our life span, but not our health span. We run out of being healthy decades before we run out of life. After we're healthy for 35 to 40 years, chronic diseases start to disrupt our lives for the next 35 to 40 years. Blood pressure goes up. Insulin resistance means a shift toward obesity and away from muscle mass. Joints ache. Plaque develops in our arteries and heart attacks occur. A vibrant libido becomes a distant memory. Acid reflux and other digestive issues happen. Brains start to slow down so we have senior moments when we walk into a room and can't remember what we're looking for.

Instead of merely managing these diseases for the second half of your life span, wouldn't you rather extend your health span as well? Can we make 90 the new 60? It won't feel that way if you turn 90 in a nursing home where you're bored and achy and miserable. That's not longevity. That is not quite being dead yet, but *living*? I have doubts.

My goal is to extend your health span so it's as close to your life span as possible, so when the time comes, your slide downhill will be super-quick and super-painless.

How This Book Came to Be: Scar Tissue and Stubbornness

I was born at Patuxent River Naval Air Test Center in Maryland in 1947. My father was an Aviation Division chief with an eighth-grade education who only had 30 days of leave every year, and my mother was a stenographer. I was raised on military bases and while my dad was hardly ever home, I had thousands of strong, tough, patriotic young men as role models instead. Men for whom duty, honor, and country meant something.

I was a smart kid, at the top of every class in school. I was so bored that I said to my fifth grade teacher, "Look, you're going way too slow. Why don't you give me all of the first semester's work? When I finish it, let me go to the library and read." She did; I knocked out the work in a couple of weeks; then off I trotted to the library. I did the same thing in sixth grade, but by then I had already read everything in our little one-room library. I was given permission to go downtown to the community library, where I sat on the floor in the stacks and read science fiction. When I ran out of fun stuff, I read the *Encyclopedia Britannica*.

By ninth grade, my father was stationed at Point Mugu and we moved to Long Beach, California. Those were happy days; I majored in surfing and girls. And with the great forward planning of a teenager loaded with more testosterone than brains, my plan was to enlist and join a good combat unit, earn lots of decorations. Then, when I turned 19, I would attend Army Officer Candidate School, get my commission, and retire as a general at 40. College had never occurred to me. I didn't know anybody who'd gone. My dad dropped out of school in eighth grade to plow the fields and support his family because his father had died. College was for rich kids.

I was so gung-ho about the army that I didn't attend my high school graduation in May, 1965. I enlisted, hopped on the bus, and got off at Fort Ord, California. I turned 18 on the machine gun range, spending that day blazing away with thousands of rounds of taxpayer-paid ammunition. Then I ran back to the barracks in the evening with the other macho guys like me. Best birthday ever!

During basic training, when I took the exams to determine my best skills, I aced almost every test. The higher-ups tried to talk me out of active service. "Look, we can send you to intelligence school," they told me. "You can go to college, we'll pay for it, you'll come in as an officer. You will do more good for yourself and us." Nah, I wanted to be a tough guy and fight. I volunteered for the infantry and then paratrooper school at Fort Benning. I was shipped off to Vietnam, and in 1966 I was assigned to the 173rd Airborne Brigade. My fellow paratroopers and I were proud to be the most lethal things in the jungle.

Until one mission, when we were dropped in the wrong place and mistakenly walked into a North Vietnamese regimental base camp. There were about 1,500 of them and 42 of us. It was a tough day. We held them off by ourselves for 8 hours until we were rescued. A hand grenade shredded my left knee; a bullet clipped across my ankle; another bullet skimmed down a couple of millimeters over my back and blew off half of the right side of my ass. I had shrapnel scattered all across my left side. I still have a piece of metal in my diaphragm under my heart. One round went through my right arm; even now, if I drop my wrist, I still can't close my fingers and if I raise my wrist, I can't open them. Two rounds hit my left arm. It took me two years to be able to almost straighten it. There were eight survivors and I was the only non-amputee survivor in the bunch.

I spent the next two years recuperating and having endless surgeries in Letterman Army Hospital in San Francisco. I wanted to get as healthy as I could. I'd always been active and was determined to keep being active. When they told me I was 90 percent permanently disabled, I became stubborn and argued. I turned to the major and said, "Sir, if I can't be active combat, there are things I can do for the team." He laughed. "Son," he said, "you're held together with scar tissue and stubbornness. Get the f**k out of here and make something of yourself."

That was the last military order I ever received. I like to think I have honored and fulfilled that order in full. And beyond.

I had bullet holes and shrapnel throughout my body. The extreme violence I'd experienced in Vietnam set me up for PTSD. I decided I never wanted to kill anyone ever again. I'd been good at that job, but I'd never *enjoyed* it. There was a difference. I went to Vietnam because my country told me it was a job that needed doing and my job was to find and kill people that my government said needed to die. But when the job was over and I was in pain every hour of the day and having nightmares about what I'd seen and done, I had to figure out, *Okay, what now?* I had no skills except blowing things up and killing people and there wasn't much call for that as a civilian. The only job I could get was at the Long Beach Naval Shipyard. The ships weren't supposed to dump sewage in the harbor, but they did. I was given a 14-foot green wooden rowboat, a 55-gallon drum, and a net. I rowed around the harbor, scooping up shit and putting it in the barrel for $1.72 an hour. Trust me on this: You've never lived until you spent a California summer afternoon in a rowboat with half a barrel of shit at your feet.

I had a lot of time to think about literal shit and the other shit in my life while rowing around that harbor. About where I'd been and where I wanted to go. Did I want to spend the rest of my life doing work like this, with other laborers whose lack of education gave them few hopes for the future? No, I did not.

I needed to get out of that boat and never harm another human being. My solution was to get an education and become a physician to help and heal people. I kept my shit-scooping day job and went to Long Beach City College at night. As soon as possible, I transferred to Long Beach State College, majoring in psychology. In between classes, I would hop on my bicycle and pedal half a dozen blocks off campus and start knocking on doors to sell Fuller brushes. After classes, I worked as a janitor in a hospital until midnight, cleaning up blood and other stuff in the morgue trays and patients' vomit and shit in the hallways. When my shift ended, I studied in the library until 2 a.m., when it closed. Then I went home to get a few hours' sleep.

My high school sweetheart, Marilyn, had waited for me while I was in the army. Everyone assumed we were going get married and I didn't have the balls to say no. In those days I wanted everybody's approval. My friends, my teachers, my government, even God. So I did what I thought everybody wanted and married Marilyn.

Our second child, who was our first daughter, Tanya, died at two weeks of age from congenital heart disease. Soon after, Marilyn became pregnant with twins, and then we had two more. I look back at that frenetic time and ask myself, *How did I manage?* I had a wife and four kids to support so I did what I had to do, all while studying and figuring out how to go to medical school. You do what you can to survive.

I didn't know any doctors growing up, or anyone who could write credible references for me. I was a lower middle class kid with lower middle class contacts. I needed an edge because there were almost 200 applicants for every medical school position in the U.S. in those days. At the college library I started reading catalogs from every college that had a medical school associated with it, starting with the schools that began with an A. It was discouraging, because I was all the way down to the U's when I finally found what I was looking for—a bachelor's degree in microbiology, taught at and by the medical school faculty at the University of Utah. I immediately changed my major at Long Beach State from psychology to microbiology, applied to the University of Utah, and miraculously got in. Once I arrived, I made sure that I was the wonder boy in those microbiology classes, so when it came time to apply to medical school, I'd have recommendations from the medical school faculty—and that's what got me into the University of Utah School of Medicine.

For the first time in my life I was surrounded by people who were as smart or smarter than I was. Bright, motivated people who'd had all the educational advantages that I did not. I was the only disabled combat veteran in the bunch. When I graduated in 1976, I wanted to be a country doctor, the only doctoring I knew. I accepted a family practice residency and learned to perform major surgeries, deliver babies, and set broken bones. I then opened my own practice in Preston, Idaho, a town with just one stoplight in its county. We were three doctors in a 14-bed hospital—the emergency room, the obstetrics' department, the cardiac care unit—*everything*. My fellow doctors and I sometimes called it pucker-butt medicine because our anal sphincters were in spasm about half the time!

I was privileged to be the first human being to touch hundreds of new lives as they were born. At other times, I was the last person to hold someone as they were leaving this earth so that they did not die alone. In between, I did everything I could to improve the lives of my patients and make and keep them as healthy as possible.

Marilyn and I stayed in Idaho for seven years. We had more children and adopted two from Korea. Marilyn's focus was children and mine was supporting our ever-growing family, but we were barely scraping by. Nobody had medical insurance. An office visit cost a whopping $9; an extended visit was $12. Many patients could only afford to pay in pigs, sheep, or chickens. We ate a lot of chicken. We three doctors were running our asses off—hospital rounds before the sun came up, office visits until sundown, and then back to the hospital to do evening rounds. I was seeing 40 people a day and was on call every third night and weekend to handle the emergencies. It was a stressful and exhausting existence.

In the meantime, Marilyn was a wonderful wife and mother and really wanted to make things work. I was doing my best to make our marriage a success even though my heart wasn't in it. I was married to my job. I have to admit I was not much of a husband or father. At the end of 14-hour workdays taking care of sick and frightened people, and four or five phone calls after midnight, I lacked the emotional resources to give my family what they needed and deserved.

If I'd been smart about trying to save our marriage, I'd have gone to a bigger city and worked a 50-hour week. Instead, foolishly on my part, we moved to another small town and a small practice in Shelton, Washington. Once again I was working incredibly hard, barely seeing my wife and children, and still not making enough money. Things became so bad that Marilyn and I decided to get divorced before we hated each other. The fault was all mine. I was not grown up enough to be married.

Marilyn soon married a great guy who was a much better father to our children than I had been. Most of what I earned went to her to take care of the kids, but I was free to move on.

In 1990, I attended an endocrinology conference and heard Thierry Hertoghe, a Belgian endocrinologist, talk about his longevity clinic in Brussels. As I listened to him discuss his hormonal and other treatments, I thought, *This is crazy. This is brilliant. This is cutting edge. This is longevity. If we could really do this, wouldn't all doctors be doing it? Something's wrong. Something doesn't fit.* I invited him to dinner and the more we talked, the more I realized that one of us didn't know what we were talking about, but I was afraid it might be me. His theories about longevity seemed to be legitimate, and I was so intrigued by what he had to say that I flew to Brussels to visit his clinic and talk some more with him and some of patients. I found out that he charged an enormous fee for his services. The total cost was fine if you were a multi-millionaire, but totally out of the grasp of the middle class. Once I got back, I spent every week making the two-hour drive from Shelton to the University of Washington School of Medicine and started pulling journal articles from their medical library until the wee hours. I found solid medical literature to support what he told me.

I realized that I'd found my true calling, even though the concept of treating people to improve their longevity, let alone longevity clinics, didn't exist in this country then. After two decades as a country doctor, I'd been sitting with my colleagues in the front row looking to make changes in medicine in the U.S. Against my will, I found myself working for state, federal, and private insurance carriers. Since they paid the bills and made the rules, I was told what tests I could order, what diagnoses I could use, and what drugs I could prescribe. I was profoundly unhappy about that change in my profession. I wanted to go back to working for the patients I deeply cared about—not the insurance companies.

But I didn't want to create a longevity clinic that only the very wealthy could afford. I desperately wanted to take these therapies to Middle America. All of my colleagues told me that I was out of my mind, that I was going to ruin my professional reputation or starve to death. They knew, as I did, that no insurance company would pay for these treatments. And they also believed that no one would to be willing to pay out of pocket for medical care.

I had to try.

I figured that if I made the costs of annual longevity treatments less than annual car payments, my patients could choose between the two. If your new car is more important to you than your body, well, you can make that choice. But if your body is more important to you than a new car, you can make a different choice.

I had a patient who heard me say that in a seminar. After a few years of coming to the clinic, she said, "You know, Dr. Mixon, I almost decided to quit your clinic this year. I was feeling so good, I figured I could find a new team and tell them what I needed. But did I want to take my decrepit body out of a newer car or drive my decrepit car and keep my newer mind and body? I'm staying here." Twenty years later, she's still coming to the clinic!

It took me more than eight years of intense study and research to come up with a viable system. I used myself as a guinea pig. I asked my friends, previous patients, and every person I knew to be testers for free—even my mother, who happily volunteered—while I was figuring out what worked.

I had to keep my full-time job as a country doctor to pay my overhead and for my kids, and money was still tight. When I opened my first clinic near Seattle in 1998, I'd worked all day in my little town two hours south, then drove up to my rented office. I couldn't afford a motel, so I slept on the floor under my desk, washed up in the public restroom the next morning, and saw what few patients I had attracted. I drove back to my Shelton practice at noon and worked until 10 o'clock at night to keep the bills paid.

I almost went broke. I did everything the advertising people told me to do—ads in the newspaper and local magazines and on the radio, but that brought in a mere handful of patients. It was pathetic. I couldn't pay the rent. I was going deeper into debt every month. I maxed out my credit cards and spent all my savings. Yet even then, when I had few patients and was drowning in debt, I still knew that the fundamental science behind my program was sound. If I had more patients, I'd be able to prove to the world that what I had created was going to work.

In a stroke of luck, Pete Talbot, a marketing expert, showed up in my office. I told him what I was doing and why. He said, "Why isn't this place full?" When I told him I didn't know what to do, Pete took over my marketing and taught me to do seminars and start a call-in radio show.

Business took off. I was able to hire staff and dig myself out of debt for the first time in my adult life. As soon as I could afford it, it was deeply satisfying to give my country-doctor practice to a young Pakistani doctor, who had recently come to America.

Many of my patients came to the clinic because they listened to me on the four-hour radio show I've been doing every Saturday since 1999. My goal has always been to keep the prices low—Longevity Medical Clinics are the lowest-cost comprehensive clinic of this type in America. I do my best to make people as strong, fast, lean, smart, and as sexy as they possibly can be. When one of my patients, an orthopedic surgeon, asked me to devise a supplement that would help his patients recover more quickly from their injuries, I developed Relief Factor to help the body decrease inflammation and pain perception caused by exertion and aging, allowing people to heal faster. It has proven to be hugely successful, as have the other supplements we sell in our clinics and online.

But the success of our clinics is local to Seattle. Most Americans and even most American doctors don't have a clue about how to treat longevity with a system that works. That's about to change!

Looking for Optimal, Not Normal

My system came together by looking at what we are when we hit our peak and are at our best. I sat down and studied the characteristics of the human body at age 25.

I categorized every part of what makes us strong, fast, lean, smart, and sexy in different organ systems, along with inflammatory and immune responses. What hormone levels do we have? Why accept lower values as the new normal as we get older?

Then I had an a-ha! moment when I realized something about *normal*. Normal isn't about how you function at your best—that's *optimal*, not normal. As you'll read in this book, normal, not optimal, is the attitude of conventional medicine in this country.

How could I take people whose test results were *normal*—the normal-but-undesired changes of aging—and shift them to optimal? Your blood pressure may be normal for your age group, but is it optimal—the best is should be for you as an individual? What is your optimal weight? Optimal bone density? Optimal strength? What should your memory and cognitive skills be like? Doing this for my patients became my clinic's North Star.

When I start working with a 70-year-old, for instance, I'm much further from that North Star than I am when treating a 50-year-old. But at the clinic, we take whatever improvement we can get and build upon it. If the 70-year-old follows the program, he'll get results. Of course, if he doesn't, he will remain the same! A lot of people want instant progress, but they aren't willing to put in the necessary time and work, and ultimately fail.

Longevity and Healthcare

I don't know of any healthcare insurance companies that cover longevity treatments. When people ask me, "Why don't you accept my insurance?" I always answer, "Your insurance doesn't accept what I do."

Our medical system is focused on acute care and fixing things when they go wrong. While doctors are incredibly successful at lifesaving treatments, it's counterproductive and unbelievably costly to *treat* disease rather than *prevent* it in the first place. It's frightening that doctors can now only spend about six or seven minutes with their patients during appointments because the insurance companies demand that they see as many people as possible during office hours. Doctors don't want to do that but most of them don't have a choice.

Insurance is for disease, yet aging is not a disease. It's a normal process. *You're not sick, you're just old!*

Worse, you're told that since aging is a normal process, your only choice is to learn to age gracefully. This is a paltry euphemism for accepting that you're getting weak, slow, fat, dumb, and sexless because there's nothing you can do about it. *Wrong!* Of course, for some people, there comes a point at which they can't do any more, but most people can do a lot more than they realize.

I Was "Old" for Four Months—and I'm Never Going Back!

I was 50 when I opened the Longevity Medical Clinic. After doing the research I needed, I slowly started taking testosterone, pregnenolone, progesterone, thyroid hormones, and DHEA, as well as a fistful of supplements. For more than 26 years, I've used all the tools possible to make the significant changes needed to give me the hormone balance of a 25-year-old, so I never knew what it's like to be old.

When my beloved second wife, Banding, wanted to get pregnant, I had to temporarily stop taking the sperm-suppressing testosterone and other hormones I'd been taking for decades. I went into male menopause overnight and found out what most 64-year-old men feel like. What *normal* for my age was. It was *awful.*

My muscle mass started to shrink. I was tired, grumpy, and depressed. My metabolism shifted toward packing on fat big-time. Instead of running three or four miles without getting short of breath, I became exhausted just going around the block. Instead of doing 60 push-ups, I could barely manage 15. Everybody in the office said, "Stay away from Jerry. He's in a bad mood."

That lasted for four miserable months. Because I'd had a vasectomy, my sperm had to be harvested for Banding's IVF procedure. I was counting the hours until that happened. The minute I got off the surgical table, I went back to my regular hormone regimen. It took six long months to get back to where I had been before I had to start the four months of being WTF-I-am-old-and-this-just-sucks phase.

What does this mean? *That your current state of health is reversible.* I'm not just saying that—I lived it. I'm not going back to *normal*-for-my-age ever again—and I don't want you to, either!

How to Use This Book

When he was elected, Donald Trump was our first obese president in decades. I fantasized that he would say to his fellow Americans, "I'm too damn fat and so are you. Let's get lean together. I'm gonna lose weight in the next four years. I want you to join me and do the same thing."

If he had done that . . . if he'd been our cheerleader and tracked his progress . . . and if people had followed his lead and lost weight, the number of people with type 2 diabetes, coronary heart disease, hypertension, stroke, and gallbladder disease in the U.S. likely would have dropped by at least half.

Since he turned down the job, I'm more than willing to take on the assignment and encourage the American population to become lean. If you follow the program in this book, you *will* become stronger, faster, leaner, smarter, and sexier.

Everything in this book is based on what we do with the thousands of people who come to the Longevity Medical Clinics, as well as what callers to my weekly radio show ask about. Week in and week out, I get asked the same thing on these same four topics: What can I do about my weight? What about heart disease? Am I losing my memory? Where oh where has my libido gone?

In Part I: I explain the basic science behind aging, the importance of hormones, why you're in pain or feel sick so much of the time, and what tests and supplements might help you reach your optimal health.

In Part II: You'll discover how to implement what you learned in Part I so you can be stronger, faster, leaner, smarter, and sexier. Together we can return you to a younger, healthier you, if you follow these three steps:

1. Discover ways to reduce consumption of excess sugar that turns into the body fat that can shorten your health span and make your life span miserable. The first and single most important thing that I want to change is for people to become lean. Excess body fat makes our bodies break down much faster than having a lean, trim body.

2. The second step is to get fit as you're becoming lean. Starting a new or improving your current exercise routine doesn't mean marathon training and it doesn't mean pain. It means finding something you love to do to move your body more than you are doing now and moving it in an efficient way. Find a fitness routine—swimming, walking, dancing—that will motivate you and make our daily get-a-move-on as much of a habit as brushing your teeth.

3. Ideally, you'll be able to use hormone replacement along with its constant monitoring. If you can afford to go to a longevity clinic that treats patients as we do, that is ideal. Your body will be evaluated to see where it's strong, and where it's not and things are going to hell. Then professionals can help you to rebuild. My clinics cost about $6,000/year, including unlimited doctor visits (with no less than an hour spent with each patient per visit) and unlimited laboratory tests (done in our own lab), prescriptions, and supplements. We prescribe compounded bio-identical hormones that are unique to your individual needs and will jump-start the process of turning back the clock. We regularly track your progress so it can be fine-tuned as needed.

If you can't get to or afford a clinic, you still have options. Ask your primary care provider or an endocrinologist to order the lab tests you'll read about in Chapter 4, and insist on trimonthly re-testing to track your progress. If your healthcare insurance pays for doctor visits and labs, even better. Armed with the information in this book, you will be an informed consumer who can discover what hormones can do for you. You don't have to passively let medical professionals ignore your needs any longer.

In Part III: I show you how to keep your life thrilling and fulfilling with less stress, better sleep, and increased passion and purpose.

Longevity means making significant lifestyle changes. In this book you'll find many ideas to fuel your body without constant eating. You don't have to spend money to exercise. Walking, hiking, and running are free. Doing yoga and exercising in your home are free. Eating smaller, healthier meals is going to save you countless dollars while improving your longevity. Toss all those fad diet books away. Suffering and starving for a month or two only makes you miserable. Also, once you give up the diet-of-the month, the weight will come right back on.

You can only climb so high in the years that Mother Nature is going to give you as your natural allotment. Your parents and your grandparents never had these choices to improve their longevity. Perhaps you can double or triple that amount of time. If you do what you're about to learn in this book, you will have the time, the energy, and the smarts to accomplish so much more in life.

It's not that difficult! But you still have to be a willing participant. If you want to be successful at anything, life is always going to be about putting in the work. Yet too often, the default response to hearing the word "work" is, *Forget it, that means* HARD WORK. My plan is *enjoyable* work. Doing something physical you love to do will get you moving. Changing how, what, and when you eat will make you feel so much better. Your taste buds will reawaken. You won't be constipated. You will get full nights of restorative sleep. You will have more energy. You will realize that moving your body feels so great that if you miss a workout day or two, you will wonder why you feel tired. You'll be so incredibly proud of yourself that you'll stick to the plan because you're being rewarded every day for the work you put into making your life better.

I start my day doing what doesn't feel like work. I get up, shave, apply my hormone creams, and take my supplements. Next, I do some squats and stretch a bit. I drop down on the bathroom floor and knock out 60 push-ups. (Doing all this only takes about five minutes.) I get dressed and eat a large breakfast. I take a brisk three-mile jog on one of the trails outside my door. I come back home and clean up a little bit. I give my daughter her morning piano lesson. She goes off to school and I go off to work. All before eight o'clock! This is my *something* part of the just-do-*something* path to longevity, because I don't ever want to go back to being Fat Jerry.

Only you can decide what your *something* is. If you want to be as weak, slow, fat, dumb, and sexless as I was, you don't need me. Live your life as you please. But if you want to be strong, fast, lean, smart, and sexy much longer than you otherwise would be, this book will provide you with the tools, guidance, and information to help change your life—and give Mother Nature the finger.

You never have to give up. You can make changes no matter how old you are. Your brain keeps changing until the day you die, but just because it keeps changing doesn't mean your belly has to keep growing!

My passion is trying to improve as many lives as I can, and that passion fuels my plan for your longevity. The reasons for staying strong, fast, lean, smart, and sexy is so you can enjoy all of the passions of your life. To be able to sing and dance and run like a child so you can marvel at your muscles doing their thing. To wake up every morning with gratitude for the wonderful gifts you are blessed with. To have the strength and courage to face any challenge, since they are what teach us to do better next time.

We live in an impatient society; everybody wants everything now. Make today your *now*. Start *now*. Start small. Every change you make is a change to build upon. There's always a way to go forward.

Let me show you how.

Dr. Mixon's Rules for Longevity

1. Anything strong enough to help is strong enough to hurt.

Everything in life is a matter of choices and degrees, so you can't expect not to have the potential for adverse effects. Your doctor's job is not to do things that have no side effects or risks—because those things don't exist—but to give you as many benefits as possible, balanced by as few downsides as practical.

2. The correct medication dose is one that's just enough do the job.

If one pill is the standard dose, taking two or three won't double or triple the effectiveness. In fact, taking more or less than prescribed could cause severe reactions or make you worse. Or dead.

3. If you don't measure, you don't know.

Taking any prescription or over-the-counter medication or supplement will alter human physiology. It's incumbent on you and your medical practitioners to know what your blood levels are and have them checked regularly. That's the only way to know if what you're taking is effective or causing some side effects. Every person has different absorption rates and metabolizing abilities.

A standard dose is something that works for *most* people but might not work for you.

4. If it hurts, don't be a hero.

Unhindered by the macho male complex, women tend to be more sensible if something hurts. They want to find out why and get it fixed. When something goes wrong with men, on the other hand, they immediately default to the Rambo complex. *Yeah, baby, me and Rambo, we're manly men! We can work our way through this!* So men tend to wait until disaster strikes, while women listen to their bodies more frequently when something is painful or uncomfortable. Pain is a sign that something's wrong, whether it's an achy tooth or a muscle that won't stop hurting.

5. Just because it's normal doesn't mean it's good.

Cognitive decline is a "normal" function of aging, but if you spend an hour looking for your car keys only to find them in the freezer, it's natural to worry that something's awry. When you're 18 and strong and fit and full of beans, you're "normal." But by 50, "normal" stinks. That's all there is to it.

6. If you try you might fail, but if you refuse to try, you're a failure.

Hockey superstar Wayne Gretzky said, "You miss a hundred percent of the shots you don't take." I constantly tell my daughter that I don't care whether she wins or loses. All that matters is that she made an honest effort. As long as you keep trying, whether it's something as simple as walking around the block for an additional five minutes every day or as complicated as learning how to fly a plane, you haven't failed. (Actually, if you fail at learning to fly the plane, it will make itself obvious in the disastrous result!)

7. For many people, willpower is great, but won't-power is lacking.

You better believe my willpower is great. When I'm tempted to do something, my immediate response is, "Sure I will!" Other times, the best answer is, "Nope, I won't have that hot fudge sundae. Ha."

Teach yourself the differences between *will* and *won't.*

8. If the brain doesn't work, the rest won't matter.

As Americans are living longer, dementia—what the CDC defines as the "general term for the impaired ability to remember, think, or make decisions that interfere with doing everyday activities"—is becoming a huge problem. You can find nomograms (diagrams showing different variables) online that statistically decipher how fast your brain is supposed to be declining with age. Are you prepared to see the results?

Improving the chemistry in your body is extremely satisfying. I like being fit. I like that I can pick my wife up and carry her around. I like being able to run down the street. I enjoy my strength and my energy, but if my brainpower fizzled, I'm done for. You *can* alter your brain chemistry no matter how old you are, and those changes will have a profound influence on how you feel and see the world. And how others see you as well.

9. How old is old? Fifteen years older than me!

My concept of what makes someone "old" has changed the longer I live. Years ago, my parents were devastated by the death of a close friend who was killed in a motorcycle accident. I remember them saying, "What a loss. He was only 35 years old." At the tender age of 13, my immediate emotional response was, "What? He wasn't young. He was 35! He was *old!* Wait, what did he have to live for anyway?" By the time I turned 35, an "old" person was over 50. When I was 50, old was 65 and then some. Now that I'm 76, 101 seems old! Anyone under 50 is a kid to me these days.

10. Value your strengths and don't ignore your weaknesses.

We've all got both. Value your strong points. Just don't ignore your weaknesses. They're not going anywhere. Work around them.

11. We all need each other.

Alone, none of us can go far in our big, overwhelming, complex world. It's one of the great joys and adventures in life to find the wonderful people to collaborate with and learn from. We all need each other, and we should all want to lift each other up to do the best we can. Inspiration is one of the most powerful forces in the universe. So many people just give up, thinking that they can't do something, when all they need is that jolt of encouragement from someone who believes in them.

12. Life is about doing the work. Decide what you want to do and do it well.

A lot of people have dreams and desires, but they can't figure out how to make them happen.

When I was working nonstop as a country doctor in Idaho, I wasn't making much money, so I signed up to work weekly at a weight loss clinic in Salt Lake City. Rather than spend 2½ hours driving each way, I got a pilot's license when I realized it was cheaper for me to buy a used 1967 plane to fly there and back than buy a new car! Fortunately, our small family house was on 40 acres of land. I walked out the front door and hopped into the plane for a 20-minute flight.

When I came home, I'd land in the pasture. Our horses would chase me up to the house and our kids would scream with laughter. I didn't have the time or the money to *not* be efficient!

13. Start low, go slow.

Everyone has to start somewhere. Always start small and be incremental in your changes—because then they will stick. Pick up the pace as you can.

Something as easy as cutting out a latte a day can help you shed 20 pounds of fat in a year. While I'm a dedicated exerciser, sometimes I'm just not in the mood to lace up my running shoes. Once I do it, though, my mind is changed. On my not-in-the-mood days, the trick is to *not* decide to exercise for 30 minutes. I start exercising and tell myself that I'm just going to do it for *three* minutes. After three minutes, I'm still going.

14. You're never too old.

Nike's slogan is "Just do it." Mine is more like "Just do *something!*" You can be 55 or 95 and feel better when you start doing *something* to improve your health and lifestyle. With that *something*, you're already on the road to changing your entire mindset. Your brain chemistry will shift gears and help you to find the determination to keep going. To take a look at the world and say, *No, the good old days are not when I was 15. Like the song says, "These are the good old days." I've never had it better. So let's take advantage of it.* The most important thing we can do is alter our outlook on ourselves.

15. You can do everything right and things can still go to hell.

That's just life—every other item on this list notwithstanding. Be prepared, because doing it right doesn't guarantee success. Just as doing it wrong doesn't guarantee failure either.

We've all heard those stories of someone's grandma who smoked a pack of cigarettes every day, never exercised, washed down her daily slab of red meat with vodka and liters of Coke, and lived without losing her marbles to the ripe old age of 102. That grandma was the poster child for doing everything wrong, yet she still somehow had the longevity we seek without doing a speck of work to earn it. Doubtless you've also heard stories (much more likely to be true) of people who did everything right—ate a healthy diet, worked out five days a week, never drank, slept for nine hours every night, and had a loving family and a great job—yet dropped dead at 42.

Life is, well, *life*. We can go at any minute. Even more reason to take care of what you have.

Part I

How Not to Age: Weaker, Slower, Fatter, Dumber, Sexless

Chapter 1

Why Mother Nature Wants Us Dead—And What You Can Do About It

Why and how do we get old?

There is no one factor that causes you to age or determine your longevity. It's not just that nightly bowl of ice cream or that you haven't worked out in months. It's not just those 15 pounds you've put on or your vitamin/mineral deficiencies. As you read in the Introduction, Mother Nature doesn't know or care about your religion, political viewpoint, wants, needs, or desires. Her imperative is survival of the species, not the individual. From about the age of 35 on, we're programmed to go downhill in many ways and are less able to heal and repair the damages of our daily lives. This to ensure that we will die when Mother Nature wants us to, so we can quit consuming resources needed by the next generation.

For most of human history Mother Nature's heartless plan worked fine. For thousands of years, the life span of humans was in the 30s. She never cared about our aging gracefully. In fact, she saw to it that aging is all about the progressive loss of grace, strength, energy, sexuality, and endurance. Hormonal production declines and takes your metabolism down with it, so you gradually grow slow, cold, fat, and sluggish while your moods go from enthusiastic to fatigued, depressed, and anxious.

Let me explain a bit of the science behind the aging process.

What Happens as We Age?

Overall Aging

Here's the bad news:

- We lose muscle, which is called sarcopenia. Starting in our mid-30s—you know that timeframe where Mother Nature starts yanking our strings into obsolescence—the average person loses 1 to 2 percent of their muscle mass each year, a figure that speeds up for seniors.
- Our cells start to poop out; the energy production within every cell in our body declines, so we have less energy overall.
- Our hormones begin that slip 'n' slide into low, lower, and eventually lowest levels.
- Our digestion becomes so sluggish that we could fly around the world and back before we'd get any blessed relief from constipation.
- Fertility levels decline. For a woman in her 40s who wants to have a baby, the risk of birth defects and stillbirths increases significantly. Somewhere before age 50, the effective fertility rates in women drop to about zero.
- Overworked muscles and thinning skin cause fine lines and wrinkles. A loss of collagen and elastin makes for sagging skin. Decades of sun exposure lead to more wrinkles, leathery texture, brown spots, and alterations to your DNA. I've had women tell me that they woke up one day, looked in the mirror, and wanted to scream because it seemed like their faces fell overnight!
- While hair is falling out and thinning on men's heads, women find it sprouting, like the third little pig said, on their chinny-chin-chins (and upper lips). In addition, by age 50, 50 percent of women have a significant degree of hair loss on their scalps.

- Our five senses diminish, so sight, hearing, scent perception, taste, and touch are less potent. This can cause balance and other sensory issues, so we're more likely to fall.

- We realize we look pregnant or have a beer gut because our fat cells have bought real estate in our abdomens—and they're not budging. We're gaining weight even when our eating and exercise habits haven't changed at all.

- Bones weaken and become brittle, so they're more likely to break and take longer to heal after injuries. Spinal vertebral discs compress, so we shrink—sometimes by several inches. Cartilage weakens, leading to drooping noses and earlobes. Feet can become longer or wider.

- Our immune response takes a nosedive, so we can stay sick for longer periods of time, and we might become sick more often.

- We can't remember the last time we had sex. Our libido is so diminished that we don't bother to refill the Viagra prescription or do something else about it. By age 50, 50 percent of men have some degree of erectile dysfunction and nearly 70 percent of women have lost interest in sex.

- We want to call a friend to say we're going to be late for lunch, but we don't remember where we put the phone.

Here's the good news:

- We can reverse or treat much of the above when we stick to the plan in this book, especially when it comes to decreasing body fat and increasing muscle mass.

- We have years of life experience, accrued wisdom, and smarts to deal with all kinds of issues when we put our minds to them.

- We can let things slide that once would have driven us bonkers. Or at least we try to. Knowing that we're closer to the end of life than to its beginning means the little annoyances are not worth fussing over anymore because you have more pressing matters to deal with—like your health!

- We're willing to listen and seek out information that will help us throw out the junk food and start eating better, and get moving again.

Reproductive Aging

Women can become pregnant and have babies for a finite period of time. Girls usually get their periods and enter puberty between the ages of 10 and 15. They are fertile for the next two decades or so, although there are exceptions. Female reproductive abilities start to decline by the mid-30s, leading to perimenopause. This makes pregnancy difficult after 40, and nearly impossible after 45. (Women who do give birth in their 40s and beyond are likely using advanced reproductive techniques.) Once a woman has not had a period for a year, she is medically considered to be menopausal, and her reproductive ability is kaput.

Men can produce sperm for reproduction for much longer, although viability declines with age. They may also have performance problems they never believed could happen to them!

Senescent or Biological Aging

Your body contains 30 to 40 *trillion* cells. Of the 200 different types of cells, senescent cells, also called senile cells, are a natural yet undesired part of aging and disease. That's why they are jokingly referred to as zombie cells. Although they refuse to die and make room for healthy replacement cells, they no longer function as a healthy living part of your body, as you'll see in the next section.

Every cell in our body is designed to survive for a specific time and do a certain job. The lining of your gut renews itself every 30 to 40 hours. Skin cells tend to live for only 2 to 3 weeks before they are replaced by new, fresher cells. Muscle cells live for three to four months, and brain cells live for years. About 10 percent of your bones are replaced every year or so, meaning that you get a new skeleton about every ten years. But, because women have lower testosterone to start with and their estrogen levels decline from around age 30 on, the replacement bone that forms tends to be thinner and weaker.

As we age, a wide variety of factors trigger changes that slowly degrade the quality of the new cells we make to replace the old, worn-out ones. A big factor in this progressive decay of aging are those annoying senescent cells.

A small percentage of cells undergo a dramatic change as they approach their programmed time of death. Rather than die and be replaced—a process called autophagy—they undergo a metamorphosis. They enlarge, become more globular in shape, and make a radical shift in their acellular communication with their environment.

A quick digression here: Every cell in your body communicates with every other cell via exosomes and acellular vesicles. These are little packets of messenger RNA (mRNA) that bud off from the cell during its healthy life span. They are then taken up by other cells as they circulate through your body. When this occurs, they can influence the activity of cells far from their site of origin. (This is one of the many ways the microbiome and the bacteria and virus load in our gut influence our health and can also predispose us to specific diseases.) All cells do this to a greater or lesser extent. It is a big part of why a healthy diet can make a profound difference in your overall health.

Zombie Cells

While healthy cells produce mRNA that enhances our immune system and promotes growth and repair, zombie (senescent) cells release inflammatory message that do just the opposite. One way of looking at them is that they do not want to die and be replaced. Instead, they produce anti-growth, anti-repair messages to keep themselves alive for as long as possible. When those anti-growth and anti-repair messages are released into your bloodstream, they inhibit repair and the growth of new tissue *everywhere* in your body. Worse, in addition to promoting the general decline of your health and vigor, they actively promote the formation of cancers and accelerate the degeneration of everything from your brain to your joints. And, like the zombies in the movies, they actively promote the creation of new zombies!

The immune systems of healthy young people quickly seek out and destroy zombie cells. The robust immune system of a ten-year-old, whose body has few zombies, will find and kill a zombie cell in less than a day. As we age, however, two bad things happen: We make more zombie cells, and our declining immune systems take longer and longer to locate and kill them. By the time we're close to age 60, the immune system needs at least two-and-a-half *weeks* to eliminate any given zombie. The result is a massively larger load of destructive anti-repair messengers flooding our system. We heal much more slowly, and become less able to grow new tissue to replace old worn-out cells. Our joints, hearts, lungs, and brains start to go downhill. Obesity, a sedentary lifestyle, smoking, and drinking alcohol—virtually every habit we know to be bad for us—accelerate the number of zombies at any given time, thanks to increased production and slower clearance.

Zap the Zombie Cells

Fret not. You can zap the zombies to improve your longevity:

- Do the opposite of everything that promotes zombies in the first place. Exercise, lose weight, avoid smoking, avoid alcohol, and avoid other bad habits your mother warned you about—all this will lead to quicker zombie destruction.

- Active muscle cells trigger zombie cell death, so the more muscle you have and the more intensely and frequently it is exercised, the lower your zombie load will be.

- Certain supplements slow the formation and reduce the zombie load to some extent. Polyphenols such as resveratrol and quercetin can be modestly effective.

- A more intense treatment is with a potent zombie-killing medication, an anti-cancer drug called dasatinib, coupled with quercetin. (Dasatinib has side effects that you do not want to play with, so you need expert advice about the most effective protocols. I've undergone this treatment as have many of our clinic patients. I know it works, but only under controlled supervision by a physician experienced in the therapy who understands and can manage any side effects. The doctors in my clinics do this routinely.)

About Telomeres

A telomere is the protein cap at each end of your DNA double helix strand. Babies are born with the longest telomeres they will have in their lifetimes. As we age, our telomeres tend to become shorter. Since every cell in our bodies lives for a predetermined period of time, when the cell self-destructs, it is replaced by a new one. Each time a cell is replaced, a few base pairs are sheared off the telomere, so it becomes shorter. When the telomere becomes too short, the open ends of the DNA are exposed to the cytoplasm of the cell and the cell dies without being replaced.

When this process was first discovered in the 1980s, scientists thought that the telomere was functioning like a genetic clock—that telomere length was the best measurement of biological aging. People with long telomeres would live longer and people with short telomeres would die sooner, right? Wrong! As usually happens, life turns out to be far more complex. There is an enzyme called telomerase that adds more base pairs back onto the DNA strand. Telomere length turns out to be a balancing act between things that accelerate telomere shortening and things that increase telomere length. Almost anything you can think of that tends to shorten life—obesity, drugs and alcohol, emotional or physical stressors, smoking, etc.—shortens telomeres. All the good stuff—weight loss, exercise, omega-3 oils, antioxidant supplements like vitamins C, D, and E—increases telomerase and hence lengthens telomeres again.

When I started the Longevity Medical Clinic, we tested telomeres on every patient and repeated the test annually to track their length. We no longer believe that the test is as predictive as we once did, and the science of telomeres has fallen out of favor for anti-aging purposes. Science moves on and we need to change our practices to reflect our newer knowledge.

What You Can Do About It: Call Mother Nature's Bluff!

Let's start with the most common myths:

1. **Myth: Aging inevitably means declining health.**

   Fact: While certain physical changes come with age, not everyone will experience significant health problems. Knowledge and lifestyle can make a difference. This book shares a blueprint for the process.

2. **Myth: Aging leads to memory loss.**

   Fact: While some cognitive decline is normal with aging, severe memory loss or cognitive impairment is not. Diseases like Alzheimer's are not inevitable, even with a genetic predisposition.

3. **Myth: Older adults can't learn new things.**

   Fact: The idea that the brain can't learn or adapt as we age is false. Neuroplasticity, or the brain's ability to form and reorganize synaptic connections, continues to occur throughout our lifetimes.

4. **Myth: Older adults don't contribute to society.**

   Fact: Many older adults contribute significantly to society, whether it's through volunteer work, imparting wisdom to younger generations, or still working.

5. **Myth: Depression is a normal part of aging.**

    Fact: Depression is not a normal part of aging. If an older person is feeling depressed, it's important to seek professional help.

6. **Myth: Older adults don't need as much sleep.**

    Sleep patterns can change as people age, but the need for sleep doesn't decrease significantly.

7. **Myth: Aging means losing your independence.**

    Fact: Many people remain active and independent well into their later years. Advances in technology and home healthcare also make it easier for older adults to stay independent.

8. **Myth: Sexuality disappears as you age.**

    Fact: Sexuality is a lifelong part of human nature. Many older adults continue to have a healthy sex life, although the frequency and nature of sexual activities may change with age.

9. **Myth: All older adults are lonely.**

    Fact: While it's true that social circles can decrease with age, many older adults have fulfilling social lives.

10. **Myth: You can't prevent the effects of aging.**

    Fact: We can't stop the biological clock, but a healthy lifestyle can significantly impact how we age. Regular exercise, a balanced diet, and avoiding smoking and alcohol can help slow the physical effects of aging.

Fight Back Against the Destructive Cycle with the Virtuous Cycle

In medicine, there's a concept referred to as a *virtuous cycle*. This is when something good happens, which then sets up another good thing, which can give you improvement, which sets up a third good thing, which sets up something which brings you back to the beginning so that things go round and round and round and get better and better as they go.

On the flip side, there's the *destructive cycle*. Being sedentary and gaining weight will launch you right into that unwanted loop of horrible occurrences. Our ability to fight disease and find and kill cancer cells before they kill us is dependent in large measure on a healthy immune response. As we age, our immune response declines, which is one of the reasons cancers are more prevalent as we get older. Immune responses and our ability to zap those zombie cells are triggered by physical activity and working your muscles. Working muscles produce more than 100 peptides or proteins, called myokines, that promote the growth and repair of everything from brain, bone, heart, and liver tissue to altering our immune response dramatically for the better.

I want you to think of muscle and fat as two diametrically opposed forces at war within our bodies. These are not cosmetic factors. I do not care if you look fit or fat. Fat is actively trying to kill you! Muscle is your knight in shining armor coming to rescue you.

Muscle and fat are far more complex than previously believed. Fat is an active, destructive gland that produces more than 80 different peptides, enzymes, and cytokines that narrow your arteries, make your brain cells die faster, and cause your joints to erode and lose cartilage, which can lead to arthritis. Fat changes your immune system so that you develop cancers and dementia, and it sets you up for diabetes.

Working muscle is just the opposite. It's putting out over 100 growth and repair factors to help you heal and repair not just muscle, but also ligaments, tendons, bones, cartilage, and the brain, heart, and lungs. Some journal articles now have the number of myokines produced by working muscle up in the 300 range, rather than the "over 100" I usually quote.

So, the more body fat we have, the faster we trot off to the destructive cycle. On the other hand, the more muscle we have, especially when coupled with weight loss, the more we can kick-start a virtuous metabolic cycle. When I refer to exercise, I don't just mean a workout or strength training once in a while—I mean, full daily activity with dedicated exercise sessions along the way. Taking the right supplements will also help give you the boost you need to keep moving.

The good news is that if you increase muscle mass, you will also increase testosterone production that in turn increases growth hormone production that in turn increases more muscle. The virtuous cycle, remember? So it's time to rethink how and what you eat so you can get back and stay back in the land of the living.

Fight Back Against "Instant Results"

One of the questions I am asked most often is, "When am I going to see results?" Of course, you want to know!

Everyone's metabolism is different. Your preexisting health issues are unique to you. If you stick to the program in this book and follow the dietary recommendations, exercise regularly as described, and take the appropriate nonprescription supplements, you will see subtle changes within a few weeks. You will become stronger, and your endurance will start to improve.

But don't expect dramatic results in the first two or three weeks. You want to be the tortoise, not the hare. Results will be slow, but they will be incremental. Be patient. After three to six months, you will start seeing significant changes. If you can work with your physician or a longevity clinic to increase your hormones, you will see results much more quickly. Bear in mind that men tend to respond quickly to a restoration of their youthful anabolic hormones. Women tend to need more time, simply because their hormone balancing is more complex, so we need to go a bit slower.

The last thing you want is to get sucked into the crash-and-burn syndrome. That's the syndrome blasted out on social media and websites with enticing headlines like "Two Weeks to Your Beach Body!" or diets that promise that you'll lose X amount of weight in X amount of time if only you eat 500 calories a day or cut all carbs from your diet or drink green juices until you faint.

Forget about dieting. Diets don't work. Sure, you can lose a few pounds quickly if you starve yourself for a week or two, but nearly 97 percent of dieters regain their weight within one year. That percentage sucks! Worse, losing fat and muscle as you will from fad diets is destructive, setting you up for sarcopenia. You also lose bone density, strength, and energy. You become weaker, tire more easily, and are less able to do the activities you once loved. Seniors stuck in a destructive cycle of inactivity don't know that getting up and moving more will give them the energy they need to get up and move more!

It took Fat Jerry years of hard work to get my program adjusted to the point when all that big belly fat hanging out there and my thunder thighs faded away. Now I have lean, hard muscle. If you lose a pound a week and keep it off, it's more like six months to a year to that bathing suit. That's the reality. The kind of reality that will keep the weight off for good.

It's a long-term commitment. For the rest of your life, you're going to be doing something different with the lifestyle shifts described in this book. Accepting that there's no magic bullet to good health and a long, healthy life is the first step in the right direction.

Fight Back Against Hype and Misinformation

I discuss this in more detail in Chapter 5 when I talk about supplements. Suffice it to say for now that fads and hype about weight loss and "fat-burning overnight" pills have one thing in common: They don't work. For every legitimate medical site debunking weight-loss baloney, there are thousands of con artists trying to sell you something "new and better" for "instant results." If any diet book had a completely successful method and if any supplement showed overnight results, no one in this country would be grimacing at the scale every week. It's hard to be an informed consumer when so much misinformation goes viral and causes harm (and sometimes even death). For many people, when one fad diet doesn't work, they move on to the next.

Don't fall for the hype. "If it sounds too good to be true, it is" is one of those clichés that tells the truth.

Fight Back Against Frustration with the Medical System

I get call after call after call on my radio show from people who've gone to their medical providers and were told, "Oh, it's nothing, you're just getting old, and need to get used to it," when their symptoms were actually serious. They call me to ask for the advice they didn't get when they should have. Sometimes this is because doctors are overwhelmed by the demands for "productivity" from their bosses. Sometimes it's incompetence, although most likely the doctors are simply following the protocols set up by their clinics. When your issues fall squarely within a clinic's specific protocols, you will get fast, efficient, cost-effective care. But if you have an issue that falls outside of the clinic's protocols, things sometimes can go very wrong. Sometimes it's a doctor's ego that prevents them from saying, "Hmm, I don't know what's going on. Let's figure it out. If we can't, I know someone who might be able to help."

That's why I do a lot of referrals for people who call into my radio show. Recently, someone called on a Saturday and said he was having surgery on Tuesday. He was reaching out three days before, asking for advice about his procedure. After I told him the basics, he asked if he should go ahead with the surgery! I said, "Well, I haven't seen your labs or your other pre-op tests. I'm assuming your doctor is a competent physician and if he recommends the surgery, you probably need it. What I'm here for is to explain to you *why* he probably thinks you need the surgery. I'm sorry he didn't explain it to you, and I wish he would have, but perhaps he was incredibly busy, so I understand why this happened."

Because I have been an overworked doctor, I know I need to give my colleagues the benefit of the doubt. There are very few evil or stupid doctors out there. Most people go into medicine because they are nurturers by nature. They want to help. More than that, they have a deep-seated emotional *need* to help.

But very few physicians work a 40-hour week. Most are running from exam room to exam room 50 or 60 hours a week in addition to night and weekend call schedules. There are limits to human endurance and enthusiasm. At some point people burn out and default to the least burdensome response. When that happens, you, the patient, get short shrift. There is temptation to scribble a prescription and move on to the next room as quickly as possible.

While this is understandable, it's the antithesis of what a physician should do. The word "doctor" literally means teacher or professor. We are supposed to teach and explain things to our patients, not just do procedures or write prescriptions. There is very little teaching you can do in a six-minute appointment in which you are supposed to decipher and guide someone through a complex physiologic/metabolic dysfunction that is human disease!

Please do not blame your doctor for our systemic dysfunction. I assure you that doctors hate the insurance-driven system as much as you do! Our medical care system was not designed by doctors. It was produced by politicians, insurance executives, and attorneys.

Many years ago, I took one of my then-teenage sons to New York City for a father-son outing. Standing at the top of the Empire State Building, I was amazed how many skyscrapers featured the name of an insurance company! All those skyscrapers were not paid for by altruism. They were bought with cold hard cash thanks to putting profits first. Ignore what the companies say in their ads and brochures. The actual standard that is followed is how little can they pay in claims while collecting premiums and staying out of court.

I remember the first time an insurance company representative came to negotiate a contract with my office when I was still a country doctor. Do you know what he said to me? "We control 150,000 lives in your catchment area. Do you want access to those people or not?" There was no negotiation possible. They controlled that many lives in my community and I could take their terms and have access to their people or not. If not, I'd have no practice and these people would have no doctors. The phrase, "We control 150,000 lives" irritated the hell out of me and still does. But that is how insurance companies work.

One of the primary reasons I quit my family practice was because I wanted to go back to working directly for my patients instead of the politicians, insurance executives, and attorneys who control the mainstream medical establishment. I wanted to be a doctor who would be of benefit to as many people as possible, to help prevent diseases, instead of treating them after the damage was underway. I wanted to do certain procedures that I know are effective, but mainstream doctors can't do, since they must follow rigid protocols. That frustrated desire to teach and help patients through a broken system is a large part of why my clinics and this book were created.

Remember this above all else: *Whoever pays the bills makes the rules.* When patients stopped paying their own medical bills, they lost control of their medical care. Equally bad, when they stopped paying their own bills, they lost track of the costs associated with their care.

Your doctor is employed by whomever pays their bills—that's the insurance carriers. Whether that carrier is a private company, a state agency, or the federal government, the payers are in charge of your care. They make the rules for you and for your doctors. They tell the doctor who they can see and how often a patient can be seen for a given diagnosis, what lab tests are permitted, and what can be charged for every service provided to the insurance carrier's patients.

We have excellent health care available in this country, but only if *you* pay for it. No one else cares about your health as much as you do. If you do not care enough to take charge of what happens to you, then no one will.

Fight Back Against Comparisons

Our concept of fat and muscle has become warped over the last 50 years. We've completely changed our concept of what a healthy human being looks like. From normal to totally artificial.

Women used to have shapely, slim bodies with real breasts, hips, derrières, and thighs. Marilyn Monroe's weight fluctuated a lot, but she had a curvy (not fat) figure that millions of women wanted to emulate. But when Twiggy became a superstar model in the 1960s, the fashion industry decided that ultra-skinny was "It," and women would starve themselves to look like her. It's become far worse over the years, as a sample size for models used to be a 4 to 6, and now it's a 0 to 2. Good luck fitting into that.

Go on a streaming service and take a good look at Arnold Schwarzenegger in *The Terminator* or Sylvester Stallone in *Rambo*. They might be superstrong, but beefy men like those two certainly are not super-healthy. I doubt they got so buff solely by pumping iron. No human being, male or female, is designed to take things to such extremes to create that kind of muscle mass.

A far better role model for a healthy male physique is someone like Johnny Weissmuller in the original Tarzan movies, or Kirk Douglas in his heyday in *Spartacus*. (Look them up if you don't know who they are.) When you watched those guys and their naked torsos in action, were they buff and toned and radiating vitality? Absolutely. Were their muscles bulging all over? No way.

But for some reason, Hollywood has taken that blown-up, cartoonish perversion of human physiology and run with it. Some movie stars are loaded with massive doses of steroids and working out to make muscles on top of their muscles and cut their body fat down to a dangerously low 8 to 9 percent instead of the normal range of 12 to 20 percent. (For men, an overall body fat of 15 to16 percent is a nice mid-range. The percentage should be slightly higher for women who have a layer of fat under the skin to provide their curves.) I recently saw an interview with Sylvester Stallone, who said his body fat was only 2.8 percent when he made his last Rocky movie. In the process of holding that ultra-low-fat range during filming, he felt awful, and had serious memory issues and fatigue. I certainly believe him. No human being is designed to carry that little body fat.

Human males are supposed to be lean and angular, not soft and rounded like four-month-old babies. Human females are supposed to have a thin layer of fat under the skin to round them out. But under that thin layer should be firm, active muscle. In my seminars, I used a photograph of a black panther, her muscles taut as she prepared to leap from a tree branch in the jungle onto her prey, as an example. *That* was a lean, sexy jungle cat. That's what we should strive for.

And when I say lean, I don't mean *skinny*. I've seen fashion models sashaying down catwalks who are so skinny you can count their ribs, but they're not exuding any kind of vitality. They're not lean—they're desperate for a meal!

Of course, we all make comparisons to others. It's just human nature. Sometimes they can be helpful. If, for example, we compare ourselves to someone our age who just lost a lot of weight and kept it off, this may spur you to believe you can do the same. Comparisons can also be self-destructive, such as when we make them to placate ourselves: *Well, I know I need to lose weight but that woman walking up the street over there needs to lose more than I do, so I'm okay*. Or, we get bummed out when a friend can eat and eat and not gain weight due to her metabolism. Then we give up because comparing ourselves to someone we'll never be like can be extremely painful.

I admit that I am sometimes guilty of comparisons that might not be ideal. I know my trim belly is pretty amazing for a 76-year-old man. It's solid and I work hard to keep it that way. But not that long ago, my wife and I were taking our evening walk on a nearby trail. Four young guys from nearby Northwest University came running down the trail toward us. They were 19 or 20 years old, with flat bellies and tiny waists, running like the wind. I looked at those guys and said to myself, "Damn, I want that belly. What I have is pretty good, but I want better." I started kicking up my exercise routine a little more and cutting back on my food intake. We'll see how well I can do! The major motivator in my life is my wife, who is 30 years my junior. If she has three extra fat cells on her body, they have never met. When we run together she is usually in front. I tell her that I lag behind just so I can watch her cute tush move when she runs. The truth is, I could not have caught up with her when I was 18. I carry too much muscle mass and she is just a lean, fierce, lovely woman. She enjoys having a firm, lean man in her bed, and I enjoy being that man! I am motivated not just by knowing how I need to improve my longevity, but by love and a healthy dose of lust to stay in shape.

The bottom line is: The only person you should compare yourself to is you, your own body, and your own habits. If you're just getting started, the most valid comparison will be with what shape your body is in now—not 30 years ago, when you could easily lose weight, run five miles a day, and go out partying every weekend and still get to work on time on Monday. You will be able to check in a month or six months or a year to compare the results with your starting point and see how much progress you've made.

Trends and fashion will change. The thing to remember is that when you follow the Longevity Medical Clinic formula, you're going to be the best version of you—the healthiest version you can be regardless of your age.

I want to remind you that the guy on the book cover is me. A 76-year-old physician, who at 50 was fat, tired, depressed, and sexless. I enjoy being the fellow kicking the clock, representing time in whatever time uses for as a tush. I am leaner, stronger, and happier than I ever dreamed of being at 50. And you can do the same things I have done.

What you are today does not have to be what you will be in the future!

Fight Back Against Your Denial

In order to take the first steps to change your lifestyle, it's time to get real and admit to some unpleasant truths you've been ignoring. I know it's not easy; I was Fat Jerry, in total denial, remember?

So many of us blame ourselves when something goes wrong, or if we're ashamed of our bodies. We tell ourselves, "Oh my God, I just ate that huge slab of cheesecake. I'm such a bad person. I'm so fat. I'll never lose any weight." This is actually a form of denial—a person telling themselves they're unworthy of trying to make changes. I'd like to see that response changed to, "So here's that huge slab of cheesecake I'm craving, I can eat it or not. Or I can eat a few mouthfuls and chuck the rest. If I do eat some, I will slowly savor what I put in my mouth because I know I will not buy it again in the foreseeable future."

Another response might be, "Well, I know that a 150-pound woman who walks or jogs one mile burns 100 calories, and there are 800 calories in this piece of cake, so I need to walk an extra eight miles today to compensate. What should I do? I know, I'll take two bites and go for an extra-long walk. No way do I have the time, inclination, or energy to walk eight miles." A healthy compromise is a healthy choice.

I can't tell you how many new patients come into our clinics and tell us they need to lose ten pounds, when their objective measurements tell us that they need to lose at least 50. These patients are making honest mistakes, because society's current concept of what's "overweight" has become warped over time. If you look at photos of Americans in the 1940s or 1950s, obesity was rare. Kids walked to and from school and rode their bikes to play with friends. Adults were more active and ate healthier diets. Junk food and microwaves hadn't been invented yet. I like to joke that the beginning of the obesity epidemic came with the invention of the TV remote control; no longer did we even have to get up to change the channels. Now, of course, you can surf online for days at a time without budging from your chair.

Clothing sizes are no longer an objective measurement. If you're a size 8 now, you would have been a size 16 back in 1958. Today's clothing manufacturers want you to think you're slimmer than you are. And if everyone you know is heavy, it's only human nature to see heavy as normal.

There is a major cultural component to this as well. My wife, who was born in China, wears American-size 00 pants and XS shirt. When shopping in China, she buys size medium! She is not considered slim in China.

Here are some worrisome facts: The heaviest groups in the U.S. are Native Americans or have African ancestry. They also have the highest rate of stroke and heart attacks. The second heaviest group are those with Hispanic ancestry. They have the second highest rate of stroke and heart attacks. Caucasians are the third highest in both fat and vascular disease. Asians are the thinnest group in America and have the lowest risk of stroke and heart attacks. Weight matters!

Fight Back Against Anyone Telling You That You Are Too Old

Before I opened my first longevity clinic and was still developing the program, my first elderly patient came to my family medicine practice. She was leaning on a walker and could barely move. It took her five minutes to get across the tiny exam room. She was in terrible shape. She told me she was 93, but when I looked at her chart, I could see she was 98. I laughingly had to remind her that, you know, my M.D. stands for minor deity, so it's a sin to lie to your doctor!

She said she'd heard rumors that I was testing out a new program. "I want what you're doing for those other people," she said with a determined look on her face. Well, I'd never thought of treating a 98-year-old woman who could barely move. Plus, I had a feeling she had limited means. "Ma'am, what I'm doing costs some money," I said as gently as I could. "And quite frankly, I don't know what I could do to help you because you're 98 years old and I've never treated anyone your age. I don't want to take your money if I can't help you, but I don't have enough money to treat people for free."

She stopped me right there. "Doctor, it's true," she said. "I don't have a lot, but I'm dying. I feel like I'm encased in concrete. I've been in the hospital five times in the last year. If we don't do something, I'm going to die. And whatever I've got left when I die, someone else is gonna spend. So why don't I spend it to see if you can help me or not?"

I didn't know how to argue with that, so I took her on as a patient, keeping costs as low as I could for her. I started by restoring seven of her hormones to more youthful levels to allow her to grow muscle and repair some of the damage that aging had done to her. The hormones we started her on were testosterone, DHEA, estrogens, thyroid, progesterone, and pregnenolone, as well as a touch of GABA and melatonin to help her sleep, and a few supplements designed to lower her systemic inflammation. She also put our advice on diet and exercise into action almost immediately. Within a year, she no longer needed her walker and was walking a quarter mile twice a day for exercise. She carried a cane on her walks in case any dogs bothered, her, but she didn't really need it. Three years later, when she was 101, she was quite proud when she came into my office. She was standing up tall, walking with no aid at all, and announced that she had just mowed her own lawn. She practically gave *me* palpitations because the concept of 101-year-old woman mowing her lawn scared the bejabbers out of me. "I hope it is a tiny lawn," I told her, "and I also hope it was a lawnmower that pulled you so you didn't have to push it!"

This amazing woman got her life back. While she didn't become strong, lean, and completely fit, she was going to the mall again and visiting her great-grandchildren. She was so proud of herself until the day she died at 103. But in those five years, between 98 and 103, instead of five hospitalizations a year, she averaged two. She was motivated because she honestly believed she was dying. I suspect she was probably pretty close when she came to see me.

Even people like her can be helped. I can't get them running or lifting their body weight. But if I can get them walking again, I count it as a win. We'll take whatever progress we can and use that to step it up to the next challenge. It all depends on where you're starting and how much effort you're willing to put in.

It is extremely gratifying to see my patients—many of whom had given up taking care of their health and were desperate for any advice and encouragement when they came for an initial consultation—transform their physical health and emotional well-being. Not only do they look and feel better, but they've learned to congratulate themselves in terms of self-encouragement and pride for their accomplishments.

Sometimes, I have to say, people think, "Start slow, go low" means "Don't go." Nope! It means you start with an achievable goal. I lived through this after I came back from Vietnam. A hand grenade had shredded my left knee and thrown mud and leaves and debris into the joint and it became badly infected. I drained puss out of that knee for the best part of a year. Learning to bend my knee again to break up the scar tissue and get it so the knee would flex to a usable degree was agonizing. Then I had to relearn how to go up and down stairs because the knee wouldn't support me on just one step, much less an entire flight.

I started low with one step. Read this correctly. I am not saying one step at a time. I literally had to start by getting my knee to carry me up one step, period. Then having mastered that, I did two and then three steps, until I could do a flight of 12 or 13 steps with minimal pain. I had to start with what I could not yet do but believed was achievable. Because when you set small goals and achieve them, then the next goal is merely the next goal. It's getting to that mindset of *You can do it* at any age. Today, I go up hundreds of steps on hikes and during our family travels, and I have no pain.

It begins with where you are today. Not where you wish you were; not where you want to be eventually. Then you set your goals for something that's achievable yet a bit difficult so that it moves you out of your comfort zone. To me, isn't that the definition of progress? Moving out of your comfort zone? If you're totally comfortable with it, you're not moving!

That's what I've always told my daughter about mistakes. During one morning piano lesson, I was trying to teach her one of those blazing fast runs in Mozart's sonatas. I played some recordings for her first. "Dad, I can't do that," she said with a crestfallen face.

"Oh, yes, you can," I replied. "You just do it about 40 times slower than that concert pianist. Let's slow it down, and when you master that, then you can do it a little faster. Speed comes with practice." Now, she can play rapid runs blindfolded to demonstrate her muscle memory.

It's the same way with exercise, weight loss, and lifestyle. You have to start somewhere, and you have to do something that is a bit uncomfortable. It should not be super-easy. You should have to think about it and put some effort into it. Then, once you've got that mastered, don't stay at that level. Pick the next step and improve upon that.

If you're not making some mistakes in any new endeavor, you're not living close enough to the edge of what you can do. Make mistakes and learn from them. Then move on to new challenges and make new mistakes next time. If you have a setback—perhaps you have to work longer hours or a family member needs you, so your workout time is curtailed—a small setback is not a total setback. Don't use it as an excuse to avoid moving forward. One of my many aphorisms for life. Don't be afraid of mistakes. Try something, make your mistakes, then learn from them and move on to new and better mistakes!

When new patients come to my clinic, I remind them that I want them to get their money's worth and I want to see them succeed. I also give them my little Yoda talk.

My Yoda talk will work for you too. It's simply: "There is no try. There is *do*; there is *not do*."

That's it! You do or you don't. In other words, there's no such thing as *trying* to exercise. You either exercise or you don't. You either control your eating or you don't. The *try*—or rather, the try and give up—is an excuse for not doing.

Only you can take responsibility for your decisions to do or not do. So be a Yoda. Write down your exercise schedule and tape it to the bathroom mirror or put it on the kitchen counter or some other visible area when you leave the house in the morning; you'll see it as soon as you come home. Better yet, make it your screen saver on your smartphone. Every time you look at your phone you will see your activity list.

That's the kind of Yoda who's gonna stick it to Mother Nature.

Chapter 2

How Suboptimal Hormone Levels Reduce Longevity

"Ugh, I'm so hormonal," is something some women say when PMS leaves them with the Three C's every month: Cravings & Cranky & Chocolate. Yes, hormones make you moody. They also get you up in the morning and lull you to sleep at night, regulate your metabolism, and give you the jolt you need to swerve away from a drunk driver. Hormones help keep you alive by telling your body what to do.

When their levels start to decline with age, as they do with every human, Mother Nature is sitting in her garden, rolling her eyes as your energy fades along with your libido and your full head of hair. Once you're too old to have kids, remember, she wants you dead, and she doesn't care how miserable you feel until the day that happens.

An integral part of the longevity program at my clinics is hormone supplementation, which is our way of sending Mother Nature on her merry way. Our goal is to restore youthful hormone levels as much as possible and give bodies more tools to work with than they would normally have at a particular age. Ideally, intervention should start *before* there are symptoms. The sooner you start, the better you're likely to respond, and the less aggressive the treatment will be.

But if your hormone levels have already taken a deep dive, don't despair. It doesn't matter how old you are. I've put people in their late 90s on hormone replacement for the first time! For men, this means getting them back to levels of a man in his mid-20s. For women, it means getting them back to levels as close as possible to their mid-20s without restarting menstruation.

The good news is you don't need to go to a longevity clinic to have hormones prescribed. The better your diet and lifestyle, the more of these hormones you'll naturally produce. But here is a warning: If the doctor you see for hormone replacement only gives testosterone to men or estrogen to women, you are dealing with someone who does not understand your needs. We evaluate, and when indicated, supplement at least seven or eight major hormones in every man and every woman we see. Men and women make the same hormones, although the levels and ratios are different for each gender.

A simple but critical fact is that testosterone is the primary steroid hormone for both men and women.

An experienced physician can safely and effectively prescribe specific hormones to raise your levels to a higher and more functional range. Remember, these steroid-based hormones function to alter your mood and perception of yourself and the world around you. Older people become depressed curmudgeons because of the decline in production of these active chemicals in their brains and bodies.

Discuss all your options with your doctor and don't take no for an answer.

The Most Common Myths About Hormone Replacement Therapy (HRT)

1. **Myth:** HRT is only for menopausal symptoms.
2. **Myth:** HRT causes weight gain.
3. **Myth:** HRT affects fertility.
4. **Myth:** HRT increases the risk of breast cancer.

5. **Myth:** All women should use HRT during menopause.
6. **Myth:** Synthetic hormones are the equivalent of bio-identical hormones.
7. **Myth:** HRT causes cardiovascular diseases.
8. **Myth:** HRT causes strokes.
9. **Myth:** HRT can cause depression or mood swings.
10. **Myth:** Once you start HRT, you can't stop.

The Major Hormones That Affect Aging

Hormones are chemical messengers in your body that send directions to your cells and organs so they function properly. There are more than 50 hormones in your body, but when it comes to longevity, you only need to know about those covered in this chapter.

You may be surprised to learn that cholesterol is the mother hormone. It is an annoyingly waxy fat that can clog your arteries and lead to all kinds of problems. But without it, we'd be cooked. Virtually all of the sex- and steroid-based hormones in our bodies are synthesized from cholesterol through a common precursor steroid called pregnenolone, which then converts to DHEA (dehydroepiandrosterone), progesterone, cortisol, or testosterone, and then from testosterone to estradiol, the primary human estrogen.

Anabolic Reproductive Hormones

DHEA

Produced by your adrenal glands, DHEA is a precursor hormone needed to make testosterone, progesterone, cortisol, and estrogens. It is an elevating hormone that boosts moods and physical activity. It makes us alert and awake.

Growth Hormone (IGF-1)

Growth hormone is released by the pituitary to stimulate growth in children. You still need it as an adult. Without adequate levels, it is harder to grow and replace older, damaged tissue, including muscle and brain tissue. It keeps bones strong, reduces visceral fat, and staves off depression, anxiety, low libido, and fatigue.

While the federal courts have held that physicians can use human growth hormone off label, several state boards of medicine have effectively restricted the prescribing of it for older patients. The rationale seems to be that use of this particular hormone to improve the strength and endurance of older people constitutes abuse of the drug. I do not see why helping older people climb the stairs in their homes or walk up a hill is abusive, but I am not a state functionary.

Body builders and professional athletes use (and often abuse) it as it gives them a metabolic advantage by making them stronger. Well, when I'm treating frail 70- and 80-year-olds, I want them to become stronger so they can get out of their chairs and move about in their homes without fear of falling and breaking a bone. It's frustrating to have politicians design the system and want to stay in control of it. Medical boards are generally political appointees, which explains a lot.

Pregnenolone

A steroid hormone precursor, as you read above, pregnenolone is produced in the brain and adrenal glands. Taking it as a supplement improves cognitive function and can reduce stress and improve sleep.

Estrogens

Estrogen is not one hormone; it is a class of hormones. Every living thing on this planet that's not a bacteria or virus seems to make some combination of estrogens. Humans make a unique mixture not duplicated by any other creature or plant.

The three types of human estrogens are estradiol (the strongest), estrones (made from estradiol in the liver and consisting of about two-thirds of estrogens at menopause), and estriol (made primarily during pregnancy). Estriol is an anti-cancer form of estrogen that we use as part of our hormone program for the majority of woman we treat.

Primarily produced in the ovaries in women, estrogens regulate female sexual development. They also affect fat distribution, brain function, circulation, blood sugar levels, cholesterol levels, bone mass, muscle mass, skin texture, and mood. That's a lot! A lack of estrogens can shift your metabolism toward fat, cause memory issues, raise your risk of heart attack and colon cancer, and make you feel out of sorts and that you are just getting *old*.

Produced in the testes and adrenal glands, estrogens are present in men, too. Men use them in their brains to facilitate verbal ability, short-term memory, and as an anti-inflammatory agent. When their estrogen levels get too low, they go through a menopause-like syndrome just as women do.

The Best Way to Take Estrogen

For decades, estrogen was only available in pill form. The problem is that we are not designed to ingest sex hormones by mouth. For a woman of childbearing age, estrogen is primarily produced in her ovaries, slowly and constantly trickling into her system during the 24-hour day. When you give a woman an estrogen pill, the entire 24-hour dose is absorbed within 20 minutes or so, hitting the liver all at once and overwhelming the clotting cascade (a series of factors that result in the formation of blood clots when needed to stop bleeding). This can result in an increased risk for blood clots in her veins and stroke or heart attack.

There is one estrogen combination that you do *not* want to take. If your doctor wants to give you CEE, conjugated equine estrogens, often sold under the brand names Premarin and Provera, immediately find another doctor. This combination increases the risk of breast cancer by 28 percent, while estrogen/progesterone therapy done correctly lowers the risk of breast cancer by about 30 percent.

I prefer to prescribe a custom compounded estrogen mixture applied as a cream. Compounding allows my doctors to prescribe a mixture of estrogens specific to each patient's unique needs. The cream allows the estrogen to be absorbed slowly through the skin over 12 hours rather than in a quick 20 minutes. By adjusting the mixture of estrogens in a cream, their concentration, volume, specific placement, and surface area where the cream should be applied, the amount of estrogen released into a woman's bloodstream is more controllable.

The same principles apply to most compounded transdermal (applied to the skin) drugs, like testosterone, for both sexes, as you'll see in the section on compounding on page 68.

One increasingly common method of estrogen application is the estradiol patch. It contains the most potent human estrogen. My objection is that there are only a few strengths of the patch available, so fine-tuning estrogen blood levels is limited. With the creams, I have virtually unlimited ability to adjust the levels at any point in a woman's cycle.

Yet another choice is the pellet implant of slow-release estrogens that is inserted under the skin and releases its drug for about three months at a time. It too prevents easy or frequent dose adjustments.

What Are Phytoestrogens?

Phytoestrogens are estrogens derived from plants. They're safe but extremely weak and ineffective because you're not a soybean—you need the hormones produced by your own body! It would take massive doses of any phytoestrogen for you to receive any benefits. I tell my patients not to bother taking phytoestrogen supplements or to use any skincare products claiming to contain progesterone. They're just a waste of money. Both real estrogen and progesterone are prescription medications, so the hype is a fallacy. Eat tofu, if you want to—my wife uses it frequently in our meals for texture and protein, but not for its estrogen effects!

Progesterone

Progesterone is produced primarily in the ovaries. Often considered to be solely a female hormone, its interactions with estradiol are the primary controllers of the menstrual cycle and pregnancy. Progesterone receptors are also present in a wide variety of tissues in both men and women. It is an essential hormone for many functions in addition to the reproductive cycle and pregnancy. Adequate progesterone levels are necessary for brain function, where it provides a sedative effect, calming stress and enhancing sleep. This hormone improves memory and cognition. It also plays an active role in libido, proper bladder function, and makes skin soft, smoothing out wrinkles.

Why Men Need Progesterone

Progesterone is found in healthy young men and women in almost equal levels. In men, it is metabolized from DHEA in the testes and adrenal glands. Progesterone receptors are found in the prostate, where it acts as an anti-estrogen. As men age and their progesterone levels fall—by age 60, most men have near-undetectable levels in the blood—the epithelial cells of the prostate tend to grow and live longer, resulting in an ever-enlarging prostate gland. When this happens, the enlarged prostate gland starts squeezing the urethra so the bladder can't be fully emptied and becomes stretched out. That's why older men often have to urinate more than usual during the day and at night. At the same time, the nerves going down toward the penis start becoming damaged from the constant stretching. This partially explains why, by age 50, 50 percent of men have some degree of erectile dysfunction along with an enlarging prostate and a stretched-out bladder. If men start taking progesterone before the prostate starts enlarging, problems can be prevented. Unfortunately, progesterone doesn't shrink the prostate once it's enlarged.

I frequently prescribe progesterone in a compounded cream to be applied to the skin for older male patients. I was the guinea pig, because this is off-label use for men. Normally, a metabolic variant of progesterone, medroxyprogesterone, is only prescribed in enormous doses for criminal sex offenders to shut down their libido, so the correct dose is imperative.

It took about six months of playing with the dosing to get the information I needed to be able to give it to my patients and track their improvement.

The Best Way to Take Progesterone

For hormone replacement, progesterone is poorly absorbed through the skin for most women, so it's taken as a pill. It can be applied to the skin in addition to orally for a simple reason: It makes the skin thicker and more elastic, filling in fine lines and wrinkles and making the face, neck, and hands look younger. I apply progesterone cream to my face and neck daily to help me avoid looking my age.

Do Estrogen and Progesterone Cause Breast Cancer?

Most oncologists practicing in the U.S. believe that anyone who has had estrogen-receptive breast cancer should never take any form of estrogen, progesterone, or testosterone for the rest of their lives, as it would be too risky and unpredictable.

If you've had breast cancer or are at a high risk for it, please discuss what you're about to read with your doctors. It is my belief that breast cancer might not be an estrogen-caused disease but an estrogen-*deficiency* disease. A woman's risk of breast cancer is lowest during the period of her life when her estrogen levels are the highest. By 40, a women's estrogen levels are dropping quickly; five years later, breast cancer rates skyrocket.

Part of the controversy about estrogen, progesterone, and cancer stems from the Women's Health Initiative (WHI) Study that began in 1991 and was halted five years early in 2002. More than 27,000 women took part in the clinical trials to see the effects of estrogen and progesterone replacement after menopause. The study was stopped when it was found to have increased the risk of strokes and heart attacks. Women everywhere panicked. When doctors stopped prescribing hormone replacement for women who'd been happily using it for years, unpleasant symptoms returned in force.

This study was flawed from day one. For one thing, many of the participants were sedentary and overweight, so they already had increased risks for health problems. Worse, the hormones given were the non-human estrogen Premarin (a contraction of the hormone's source: pregnant mares' urine) and Provera (a synthetic progestogen, but not actually progesterone). Astonishingly, the group that took only estrogen did *not* have an increased risk for breast cancer! Yet that data was lost in the panic.

A decade later, the same group who originated that botched study reviewed the data again, because European studies had shown that Provera increased the risk of breast cancer by 67 percent. When they redid the data, they removed all the women who'd been given Provera from those who only took estrogen. Here's what they found: In women who took estrogen, heart disease dropped by about 40 percent. Stroke levels remained the same, although blood clot rates in the legs went up but didn't cause strokes. Colon cancer declined by almost 40 percent. Hip fractures dropped. Breast cancer diagnoses went *down* by almost 30 percent. Deaths from all causes were lower in women who received the estrogen without Provera. The European studies showed that non-synthetic progesterone did not raise the risk of breast cancer. In fact, in women who have a progesterone-sensitive breast cancer, it slows the growth of many tumors by about 50 percent.

Several smaller studies have shown that the danger from estrogen with breast cancer wasn't from the estrogens already circulating in a woman's system. The danger was from the estrogens *produced by the cancerous tumor* itself. When the tumor is removed via lumpectomy, mastectomy, radiation, and/or chemotherapy, its cancerous estrogens are removed with it. Women who already had breast cancer were given estrogen and followed for several years. The results showed that they had a 35 percent lower cancer recurrence than the women who took no estrogen. Those figures were congruent with the re-sorted date from the WHI study.

Our clinics treat many breast cancer survivors, and we carefully explain the pros and cons of estrogen, progesterone, and/or testosterone supplementation. Most physicians don't know that in a 20-year-old woman, the primary sex hormone in her system is testosterone, not estrogen. Her testosterone is at levels two-and-a-half to three times higher than her estrogen at that age. Estrogen is what allows breast tissue to grow during adolescence. Even then, a woman's peak estrogen load is still a third of her testosterone load. The testosterone protects against breast cancer, and although levels drop as women age, it still lowers the cancer risk.

Let me give you some perspective on men's and women's hormone loads. (Bear in mind I am using the values reported by LabCorp, the world's second largest commercial lab.) An 18- to 20-year-old man will run a total testosterone level between 800 and 1,200 ng/dl (nanograms / deciliter). A woman of the same age will have a total testosterone of 70 to 80 ng/dl. By age 60, a man's testosterone will have declined to 200 to 250 ng/dl and a woman's will only be running 15 to 30 ng/dl. Look closely at that. A 60-year-old man is still running levels significantly higher than a young woman.

Next, factor this into your mental picture. The 18-year-old woman's estrogen is only about 30 to 35 ng/dl. The young man's total testosterone and estradiol are 800 to 1,200 ng/dl testosterone, and 3 to 6 ng/dl estradiol. The woman's testosterone is 75 to 80 ng/dl and estradiol is 30 to 35 ng/dl. The old man is still higher in total hormone load than the young woman. Men are the hormonal ones, not women! But being hormonal means men are protected by their higher hormone loads from many of the common deficiency symptoms, such as depression, anxiety, fatigue, and dementia. Women suffer from all of these at much higher rates than men.

Raising an older woman's testosterone to more youthful female levels will often increase her sex drive, improve her confidence, boost both her physical and emotional energy, alleviate depression, and reduce anxiety, in addition to making her physically stronger and more energetic. As long as it is coupled with proportionate estradiol and progesterone levels, we see very few adverse effects in our practice.

Testosterone levels in women don't get much attention. Dr. Rebecca Glaser, a prominent breast cancer surgeon at the Millennium Wellness Center in Dayton, Ohio, and an expert on testosterone in women, has published many studies on hormones and breast cancer. In one of her larger studies, women who received intermittent testosterone therapy lowered their breast cancer risks, and those who took testosterone every day had even fewer risks. In another study of women with active breast cancer, Dr. Glaser put pellets of testosterone and the aromatase-inhibitor drug, Arimidex, in the breasts, around the tumor, to test if an aromatase inhibitor would improve their situation. (Aromatase is a protein in fat that converts testosterone to estradiol; an inhibitor prevents it from doing so, and in that way it prevents the breast cancer from making its own estrogen.) The cancers shrank dramatically.

These studies are what led me to believe that breast cancer is an estrogen-deficiency disease. By the age of 50, when estrogen levels are down about 50 percent and progesterone down about 70 percent, your breast tissue is saying, "Gimme, gimme, gimme that estrogen! I need it! I need it now!" So in some women the breast tissue seems to undergo a mutation to make its own estrogen, but the mutated tissue is no longer healthy breast tissue; it's growing like mad and producing its own estrogen. That's why women with breast cancer are often told to take an aromatase inhibitor to block the estrogen, but there's no drug that can block just a tumor. To block estrogen production in the tumor, we block it everywhere in the woman's body. The lack of estrogen ages women horribly. There's memory loss. Their bones become thin and break. Their skin ages seemingly overnight, joints and muscles ache, and moodiness sets in. On the other hand, they are alive. I would like to see Dr. Glaser's methodology more widely tested. With no supplemental estrogen, the risk increases for heart attacks, strokes, osteoporosis, fuzzy thinking, depression, and fatigue.

Bear in mind that if your oncologist works in a clinic or hospital, they must follow the established protocols of that institution or risk censure and possible loss of medical licenses. The standard of care for breast cancer in the U.S. is applied with great precision, consistency, and excellence. That standard protocol is to rarely prescribe estrogen in any form for any woman with breast cancer, and aromatase inhibitors can be prescribed after intense treatment (surgery, radiation, and/or chemotherapy) for up to five years for certain cases. It's hard to criticize that except that I believe the standard protocol is deficient.

One of the similes I have used for years is that doctors conceive of themselves as a herd of grazing herbivores, being circled by predators with law degrees, and everybody is afraid to get out on the edge of the herd where they might get picked off by the lawyers. Staying in the middle of the herd is a great way to stay out of court, but it's not the way to provide cutting edge medicine. Sick people die or they're ready to give up by 60 because they don't think there are any treatments that can help them feel better.

In our clinics, we face this all the time. If a patient's oncologist has hesitations, we send the doctor copies of the medical journal articles we refer to and let the oncologist discuss the findings with the patient. We've had physicians and oncologists change their minds once they read the literature. They simply hadn't been familiar with it. But if the oncologist is adamant that they want to do what they want to do and we want to do what we want to do, it's up to the patient to decide. It's her body and her life. Women are needlessly suffering when a viable alternative is there to explore.

Testosterone

Made in the testes in men and in the ovaries and adrenal glands in women, testosterone is the primary sex hormone for both sexes. Many people think the primary sex hormone is estrogen for women, but it's not! As noted in the previous section, a 20-year-old woman has two-and-a-half to three times as much testosterone in her system as she does estrogens, while men have *ten* times more testosterone than women.

Women think of themselves as hormonal because they spend much of their lives dealing with the hormones that lead to a monthly menstrual cycle. But, as I've said, men are actually the hormonal ones—their testosterone levels cycle twice daily, peaking at sunup and sundown. That's why many young men wake up each morning wanting sex, and again in early evening after dinner.

Optimal testosterone loads make men and women more self-confident and feel strong and positive. They build muscle and bone mass so they are stronger and keep libidos active. Too much testosterone, on the other hand, can cause side effects: aggressiveness and mood swings, bulked-up muscles, lowered sperm counts, excessive hair growth, and insomnia. A testosterone decline in men and women results in depression, digestive disorders, fatigue, increased anxiety, low sex drive, hot flashes in women, and fat gain.

Testosterone and Muscle

When patients tell me they're fatigued during the day, that is a clue that they either have a hormone disorder (perhaps thyroid) or are weak and sedentary. As we age and our anabolic hormone (especially testosterone) load drops, it becomes harder to make muscle. You have much less of this hormone than when you were younger, but what you've got is still there, so you want to take advantage of it as much as you possibly can.

There are several supplements that can raise testosterone levels in men and women from 12 to 20 percent. Those most commonly used are fenugreek, ashwagandha, zinc, magnesium, and ginger. But let me give you an example of how that is less than what we want to achieve. A 60-year-old man will have a total testosterone level of about 200 to 250 ng/dl; a 20 percent increase would bring him to about 240 to 300 ng/dl. The goal in the clinic is between 700 to 900 ng/dl. While supplements do raise testosterone a bit, prescribed compounded creams are a far better alternative.

Longevity clinics or doctors who prescribe and monitor testosterone supplements can raise levels by about 400 percent. If you can't get a prescription, a 12 to 20 percent increase thanks to an over-the-counter supplement isn't insignificant. It might make some difference in your ability to increase your muscle mass, burning more calories and boosting your metabolism, which will make you a little stronger. When you're stronger, you won't get as tired because strong muscles don't fatigue as easily as weak ones do.

About Statins and Testosterone

Statins are frequently prescribed to lower cholesterol as well as the risk of heart attacks. In studies showing the risk of death for men over the age of 60 with diabetes, statins lowered this risk, but testosterone lowered the risk more than twice as much as the statins did. Drugs like the PDE5 inhibitors, Viagra and Cialis, lowered it dramatically more than testosterone. Yet every cardiologist I know prescribes statins first.

This is yet another reason why men and women need to know about their hormones. If you're worried about your cholesterol or developing heart disease, speak to your doctor about options other than statins.

How Testosterone Helps with Digestion

Have you ever thought that your gut has muscles? Most people don't. Until something goes wrong!

When you're young and have a lot of testosterone, your diaphragm muscles and peristaltic muscles in your gut are strong, so when you swallow food or liquids, they smoothly move through your digestive system. As those muscles become weaker with age, people start having swallowing problems, choking on water, plus acid reflux and constipation. Factor in any excess visceral fat that drives up the pressure inside your abdomen that can lead to gastro-esophageal reflux because your peristaltic muscles aren't working as well as they used to.

When testosterone levels go up, digestive problems often go down, especially in men.

Hormone Replacement

Perimenopause and Menopause

"The joys of perimenopause?" my 48-year-old patient Adrianna said to me sarcastically. "Let me count the ways. Hot flashes that are totally unpredictable—like it's my own personal summer except, um, it's *winter.* I'm tired all the time, but I still wake up every night at 2:47 a.m. No matter how exhausted I am, I'm tossing and turning for at least an hour before falling back to sleep. I get brain fog at work and can't concentrate. My husband is pissed because I'm pissy or depressed half the time. The thought of sex is about as enticing as open-heart surgery, which I probably need because sometimes my heart feels like it's gonna beat itself right out of my chest. Besides, sex hurts when it shouldn't because I'm drying up down there."

She leaned back and smiled and we both laughed. "You forgot about your hair thinning and your skin getting so dry it's flaking off," I said.

"Dang, how could I have missed that?" She laughed again. "Yeah, I know it's a lot," she added, "and not everything happens every single day. Doc, this just sucks. It all just makes me feel *old.*"

Perimenopause hit Adrianna with a bang. While it is often described as the two- to three-year period before a woman's last menstrual period, who knows when that's going to be? It could be at 45 or 55. I define perimenopause as the time when women start having hormone deficiency symptoms and/or their periods start becoming irregular. We know that hormone levels peak when women are in their late teens to early 20s and then they stabilize. There's not much change until around the age of 30 and levels start to decline. How much they decline depends on how robust the levels were. Most women start to notice slight changes, such as erratic periods, mood swings, sleep disruption, in their mid- to late-30s.

A woman is menopausal when she has not had her period for a full year.

Perimenopause and menopause can be excruciatingly difficult for some women to manage. Not only are the physical symptoms affecting their quality of their lives, but hormonal decline means the end of fertility.

Childbearing is another complicating factor that has led to issues in modern life. Birth control pills are combinations of estrogens and synthetic progestogens. They trigger feedback loops that result in your own body making less of the hormones you need. But you do not recognize the problems that the artificial hormones in the pills are adding to your system. The positive use is for those who do not want to become pregnant when they're fertile; the negative effect is that deciding to stop taking birth control pills can result in a sudden and dramatic onset of menopausal symptoms.

The standard of care for many doctors is to prescribe hormone replacements of estradiol and progesterone at the lowest level for the shortest amount of time to mitigate symptoms. This certainly helps the hot flash problem, but very low levels won't make a dent in health problems down the road. What I'm looking for is how well a woman is functioning and what her symptoms are. Generally, when hormone levels hit that bottom third of the so-called normal range, most women will have some of what Adrianna experienced.

If intervention can come earlier, then women won't have many of the perimenopausal symptoms because their hormone levels won't drop. My wife Banding, who just turned 47, should statistically be perimenopausal, if not close to menopause. But she started supplementing her pregnenolone, DHEA, estradiol, progesterone, and testosterone when she was in her early 30s. Her levels remain those of a 25-year-old. Over time, she has slowly needed to increase her hormone supplementation. Her body is still functioning as it did 20 years ago—except the hormone replacement has functioned as a contraceptive. When she wanted to get pregnant at 34, we had to stop her hormone replacement to allow her to ovulate. After she finished breastfeeding, we put her back on her hormones and again restored her 25-year-old endocrine support. Now, at 47, she has no perimenopausal symptoms, her skin is as smooth as a young woman's, her breasts do not sag, and she jumps rope at a furious pace and runs like the wind. When we discuss if or when she will go through menopause, she says that she is happy to continue menstruating monthly to avoid the hormone deficiency issues her friends are experiencing.

By the age of 50, the average woman has lost 50 percent of her estrogens; estradiol levels will not reach zero until age 75 on average. When levels are down by 30 to 40 percent, tiny amounts of supplements to boost them up should begin. The same is true for progesterone. The reason menstrual periods become irregular and stop at menopause is not due to estrogen, but because of progesterone levels that drop faster than estrogens.

If you are perimenopausal and your periods are becoming irregular, you can choose to keep your hormones at a youthful level with all those benefits, but you will continue to menstruate for the foreseeable future. We can let your periods stop, and give you supplements with some estrogen and progesterone, but not enough to keep you menstruating. You will avoid hot flashes and other symptoms but will not have the full youthful hormone support of those hormones. My wife has opted to maintain full support since being lean and strong is important to her. Other women may make different choices. The right answer is what is right for you.

Even if you are menopausal, your levels can still be returned to as close to youthful as possible, short of restarting your period. Most of my patients tell me one of the few good things about getting older is not having to deal with monthly bleeding, so we tweak their medications and supplements to whichever levels make them most comfortable.

I also prescribe testosterone to almost all my menopausal patients. Their stress levels diminish and they can tolerate life's stresses better, have more self-confidence, and sleep more soundly. Menopause-related anxiety and depression (not long-term clinical depression) can diminish and even go away entirely as testosterone is an anti-depressive hormone. Glandular tissue in breasts starts to redevelop and grow again, making breasts firmer. Their youthful libido often returns. (Although this can be a problem when a heterosexual woman wants to resume her sex life but her partner is one of the 50 percent of men over 50 with erectile dysfunction. Time to jump on his issues too, so they can both jump into bed!)

Are there contraindications for women taking testosterone? Remember Rule #1: Anything strong enough to help is strong enough to hurt. Regular monitoring is needed, at least every three months. One common reaction is the growth of more facial hair that can be permanently removed by laser. Facial hair growth is usually a result of unbalanced testosterone to estradiol ratios. Many women find that using progesterone cream on their faces and necks blocks hair growth and gives them smoother, more elastic skin. The pay-off usually far exceeds any minimal side effects. I have read about women on testosterone therapy getting a deeper voice or acne, but I have *never* seen this with the thousands of our female patients. I suspect that they were not given a well-balanced estrogen/testosterone level by whomever treated them.

Male Menopause

Twenty-five years ago, we thought that men didn't need much estrogen—only testosterone. Men with elevated estrogen levels were given low-dose estrogen blockers. Then we found out that not only do they need testosterone, but they also need progesterone and some estrogen, too. Hang on a minute—if they need that, what's happening to men with low or high estrogen? Well, it turns out that if men get too much testosterone, they may become aggressive, and if their estrogens go too low, they develop brain fog, memory problems, depression, and become irritable. Sound familiar? Welcome to male menopause!

Aggressive and cranky are not a good combo for anyone. Higher levels of estrogens along with testosterone are needed. They not only reduce anxiety and depression but help start to fill male breast tissue out a bit to diminish what's unkindly referred to as "moobs," or man-boobs. Let me address that aggression issue. If a man was a well-socialized citizen at 20, moving his testosterone levels back to that range will not make him overtly aggressive. He will still be the well-socialized guy he was in his youth. If at 20 he was a bar brawler, then I will moderate his testosterone a bit to avoid that issue.

Some men are sensitive to their hormone levels; others are oblivious to day-to-day changes. Therapy needs to be customized for each person by a knowledgeable physician. I often get calls on my radio show from men who want me to tell them how much of a given hormone they should tell their doctor to prescribe. My answer is always the same. If your doctor needs you to guide them in prescribing, you have the wrong doctor for this issue. Find someone like the physicians in my clinics who have years of knowledge and experience in the field.

A six-year study on male hormone levels and aging conducted in the Chianti region of Italy looked at blood levels of three anabolic hormones: testosterone, IGF-1 (growth hormone), and DHEA. The youngest men in the study were 61 when they started and the oldest were 80. If you do a six-year study with people in that age range, some are going to die due to aging and diseases. What the researchers found in the surviving study participants was that if they stayed above the 25th percentile ranking for the blood levels of each of the three hormones studied, for the entire six years of the study, the death rate was very low. If any one of the three dropped below the 25th percentile, the death rate doubled. If any two of them dipped below the 25th percentile, the rate doubled again. If all three were below the 25th percentile, 70 percent of the people were dead by the end of six years.

What does this mean? For my patients, it means that we monitor all three of these anabolic hormones every three months and make adjustments as needed to keep their levels in the mid-range of a healthy 25-year-old. We *never* allow any of them drop to the bottom 25th percentile of normal.

So why are doctors so loath to supplement with these hormones? Because the short-term studies don't show increased survival. If you do a three-month study of women on testosterone, the women may feel a lot better, even if the doses they're using are minuscule. That's not enough time to track much-needed and accurate results. Studies, especially long-term ones, are expensive. If you're going to recruit 500 women, you're talking about a $500,000 study for just three months. What's needed is a long-term study that follows a significant number of women for ten years. That's not feasible in our fragmented medical care system. In clinics like mine, on the other hand, we follow our thousands of patients for years and carefully track the dramatic changes and progress in their health and well-being.

About Compounding Pharmacies and BioIdentical Hormones

"I just saw my gynecologist, and I told her I wanted to talk about bioidentical hormones," one of my new patients said. "She told me, 'Oh, we don't believe in those.' I asked her why not and she told me they didn't trust the compounding pharmacies, and that was that."

This is something I've heard countless times and it's infuriating. Bioidentical hormones are exactly the same hormones your own body produces, so any doctor who says they don't believe in them doesn't believe in his or her own body! I wish these doctors realized that, according to the FDA, two-thirds of the CEE estrogens prescribed in the US are found only in equine species. Since the 1950s, the standard of care for menopausal women has been to recreate the hormone balance of a pregnant horse in a non-pregnant human woman. Perhaps human females should have human female hormones. Don't you think?

I do understand why compounding pharmacies are dismissed by many mainstream doctors. First of all, doctors need to have a better understanding of pharmacology and the physics of medical absorption. When prescription drugs are pre-prepared, the dose is allegedly accurate. When you write a compounding prescription, however, you have to tell the pharmacist what base (the cream or vehicle itself) you want from a dozen different bases. Some bases are better absorbed than others. Some are hypo-allergenic, while others are highly scented. Then, you have to specify how much of this drug goes in this base and its rate of absorption over which surface area and when. It takes months of training to get doctors in my clinics to be able to prescribe compounded hormones correctly.

Yes, there have been compounding pharmacies that really screwed up. They aren't regulated to the extent that the big pharma companies are since they do not manufacture drugs for interstate trade. The head pharmacist of New England Compounding Center was convicted in 2017 after his pharmacy sold injectable steroids contaminated with a fungus that killed 64 people and infected 793 more. That was very scary and totally avoidable.

I require our compounding pharmacy to send out 10 percent of every batch it makes to an independent lab to evaluate and test for purity and concentration. When you're looking for a compounding pharmacy, ask the pharmacists how often they test their products and what percentage of the products are tested. If they balk at answering, head for the door and don't look back!

Anabolic Digestive Hormones

Insulin

Glucose, or blood sugar, is the basic fuel we burn to stay alive. It is the primary energy source for your body, just like gasoline fuels most cars. Burning glucose releases both chemical energy in the form of ATP and waste heat. (That heat is why we are warm-blooded creatures. We can keep moving when it gets cold, unlike snakes and other cold-blooded critters.) Muscle is a high-energy-consumption tissue, so it burns a lot of glucose to let us move, run, jump, lift, and dance. In the process, it generates a lot of heat, which is why sweating when we exercise helps us cool off.

There's a critical difference between humans and our cars, however. In a gasoline engine, the gas is transported in fuel-impervious tubing, so it doesn't burn anything until it gets where it's needed for combustion. In our bodies, that fuel is transported through living tissues, arteries, and veins to every part of our body, not a combustion chamber in an engine. Its burning, or glycosylating, can result once a healthy liver has been replaced with so much scar tissue that there's no room for the good tissues to grow.

Fatty liver syndrome is the deposition of fat within the liver, often due to either alcohol exposure or simple overweight or obesity. It is usually triggered by insulin resistance and the resulting obesity, and as such is a precursor to type 2 diabetes. It was first recognized in alcoholics, who would get fat infiltration along with their livers' scar tissue.

Non-alcoholic fatty liver syndrome is a newer lifestyle condition. When I was in medical school, it didn't exist since obesity was rare. In my high school graduating class of 1,000, only one kid was obese. Everybody would say, "Shh, don't say anything. It's probably his glands."

The fat in the liver is not *causing* diabetes. Instead, it's an early sign that you are headed in that direction. The liver is being infiltrated with fat because there's nowhere else for it to go. The less fat in your body, the more quickly non-alcoholic fatty liver disease can be reversed.

Think of insulin as a pro-fat chemical. The more we produce, the more fat we pack on. Accumulating excess fat is a warning that you are heading toward type 2 diabetes, a dangerous disease that can cause strokes, heart disease, kidney disease, and circulatory problems, leading to amputation, blindness, and death.

When a new patient arrives at the clinic, we give them a high sugar load to eat or drink. Then we check their insulin and blood sugar levels 30 minutes later, when they're at their peak. We often find that people with significant insulin resistance will have blood sugars of 150 to 180 (up to about 130 is the normal range) and insulin levels of 150 to 180 (under 50 is the normal range). These people are producing massive amounts of insulin, yet their sugars are way too high because they're so insulin resistant. If we can intervene at that point with our program, we prevent them from becoming diabetic. If not, they are at grave risk for becoming diabetic.

What's terrifying to doctors—and what should be terrifying to all of us—is that, according to the CDC, one in every three Americans will become diabetic during their lifetime if we don't make significant changes to what we eat and to our sedentary lifestyles. Type 2 diabetes has become so prevalent that there are disposal containers for needles in the bathrooms at many public venues so visitors can safely discard those used for insulin injections.

Fortunately, type 2 diabetes and insulin resistance can be reversed, but only when you add more glucose-burning muscle and when you change how, what, and when you eat. If you avoid high carbohydrate loads, insulin will still be released to manage the glucose in your bloodstream, but the peak is much lower, and your body will be able to drive it into the cells where it can be burned as it's coming in and not resisted to be stored as fat.

"Curing" Type 2 Diabetes

Phil was 64 and had been a type 2 diabetic for 30 years. As the years passed, his diabetes required more and more medication to keep his sugar levels under control. Three years ago, he started giving himself insulin injections. After he heard me talking on my radio show about type 2 diabetes, he came to our clinic. I was pessimistic about getting him off insulin because his disease was so long-standing, and it was unlikely that his pancreas could produce enough insulin even if we were successful in reducing his insulin resistance and increasing his sugar burn rate. We agreed to try our best.

My team started by raising his anabolic hormones (testosterone, DHEA, and pregnenolone) to youthful levels. He started a progressive exercise program designed to increase both his aerobic capacity and his strength and endurance. He lost 45 pounds of fat and added 11 pounds of muscle. As he continued to improve, we were able to reduce and then eliminate his diabetes medications, one after the other. Finally, after a year, he was able to stop taking all of them. Phil now has an A1C (the percentage of red blood cells that have been damaged by glucose, your blood sugar) in the range of 5.6, takes no medication, and said he has never felt better in his life. He did get angry at the physicians he'd seen for the past 30 years who never tried to help him with his diabetes; they settled for "managing" it. I reassured him that they were doing exactly what is considered the "standard of care." Diabetes has long been considered an incurable disease. Phil was the first person who'd been insulin-dependent and sick for three decades that I was able to get off all diabetes medication.

We often encounter patients whose insulin resistance and limited pancreatic insulin production have moved them to use oral diabetes medication. When we test their degree of insulin resistance and insulin production, we usually find that about 70 percent of them have the potential to reverse their disease and get off medication. There is a debate among physicians about whether these successful people can say they are cured or simply in remission. The remission boosters say that if or when patients return to their previous lifestyle, they will again become overt diabetics. Perhaps. When their blood sugars are all within the normal range and they no longer need medications to keep them there, I consider them cured. Semantics aside, there are a fair number of former diabetic patients in our practice, and I consider their successes big wins!

Energy/Sleep Hormones

Like everything in biology, amounts and ratios are everything. Not enough causes problems; too much causes different problems. There is a sweet spot for every hormone for every condition.

In general, the issue with aging is that almost all of our hormones progressively decline. As that happens we lose the benefit of that hormone's multiple activities within our bodies. Too much and too little will both keep us from optimal functioning. Too little usually happens with "normal aging." Too much is usually either a function of a doctor who is not expert in this field prescribing more than you need, patients self-medicating, or the presence of a hormone-producing tumor. In every event, Rule #2 applies: The proper dose is just enough to do the job.

Adrenaline

Adrenaline is our feast-or-famine, fight-or-flight survival steroid hormone. It is automatically released by the adrenal glands, so you can't control how much floods your system when your body perceives danger or stress. Your adrenals automatically spring into action even if it's something as minor as your dog suddenly barking loudly or the phone ringing in the middle of the night. They control heart rate, blood pressure, respiration rate, sweat, and blood flow so your muscles are primed for you to run or fight for your life to get out of danger.

Cortisol

Cortisol is the most potent anti-inflammatory chemical hormone in your body. Like adrenaline, cortisol is also produced by the adrenal glands, and both are released when needed in a fight-or-flight response. Often referred to as the stress hormone, cortisol has several additional functions. It is part of your body's 24-hour circadian rhythm that gets you up and out of bed in the morning. It tamps down anxiety. If, for instance, you fall and twist your ankle, there's an initial burst of fear and anxiety. Cortisol is protective and proactive, and will calm you down so you can figure out what to do. It is your body's own anti-anxiety, anti-inflammatory drug.

This makes cortisol a mixed blessing. While it has potent mellowing and anti-inflammatory effects, too much of it over time can thin your bones leading to osteoporosis; trigger cataracts in your eyes; thin your skin; make your muscles weak; shift your metabolism toward fat production; and raise your risk of both infections and cancers. If you take this steroid as a supplement, you can get any of these side effects.

So, while fear, anxiety, and pain trigger cortisol release, this can be mitigated by supplementation with optimal levels of testosterone, estrogen, progesterone, pregnenolone, and DHEA to help reduce stress and improve moods.

Melatonin

Released by the pineal gland in your brain and working in tandem with cortisol, which gets you up in the morning, melatonin is what gets you ready for sleep. That's why it's often called the hormone of darkness. (That is darkness as in the absence of light, not the presence of evil!)

For more information about melatonin, see page 275 in Chapter 12.

Mood Hormones

Dopamine, Serotonin, Endorphins, and Oxytocin

Your brain wants you to feel good, so it sends out neurotransmitter hormones to flood you with feelings of pleasure:

- Dopamine is our pleasure and reward hormone. It triggers dependence on addictive drugs, but also causes us to become addicted to our loved ones. When people in romantic relationships get dumped, their brains show the same response patterns seen with withdrawal in drug addicts, explaining why love and addiction are closely related in our brain chemistry.
- Serotonin and endorphins are our happy, euphoria hormones.
- Oxytocin is a fascinating hormone that we use often in our practice. Oxytocin makes us view the world through love-colored glasses. Gazing into someone eyes, skin-to-skin contact, and sexual arousal all trigger oxytocin release. The most profound oxytocin triggers are nipple stimulation and orgasm. When a woman breastfeeds her baby, the child's suckling triggers oxytocin release in the mother. This hormone is released with every feeding, usually about every two hours, and is repeated day and night for months, triggering an oxytocin bond between nursing mother and child that lasts a lifetime.

Sexual arousal triggers oxytocin and orgasm triggers a big burst of the hormone. Remember your first great love? You two were likely having sex every chance you got whether it made sense or not. Your brain was flooded with oxytocin. You were unable to see any flaws in your lover. They were your soulmate, sent from heaven just for you, your cosmic other half that made you complete. After a while, the constant sex became less frequent, and your oxytocin levels dropped to more moderate levels. Suddenly you realized that this person was just a human being with some flaws and shortcomings. As your oxytocin levels fell, the ability to see things in a more realistic manner was restored to your brain.

We prescribe oxytocin to long-term couples who've drifted apart and need to rekindle their emotional bond. We also use it with PTSD survivors to help them stop focusing on the negative and see the positive side of life again. It is administered via a nasal spray or as a mucosal lozenge prepared by our compounding pharmacist.

For more information about endorphins, see page 147 in Chapter 6. For more information about oxytocin, see page 229 in Chapter 10.

Metabolic Hormones

T3 and T4

The thyroid gland, located in the base of your neck, produces two main hormones, triiodothyronine (T3) and thyroxine (T4). Overseen by the pituitary gland in the brain, it is responsible for regulating your metabolism. In addition, your body needs to ingest iodine to make the thyroid function properly.

When the thyroid is overactive (hyperthyroidism), it makes too much thyroid hormone; when underactive (hypothyroidism), there is too little. These conditions are very common, but because there are so many symptoms (weight gain or loss, feeling too cold or too hot, lack of energy, sleep disorders, dry skin, thinning hair) that can have other causes, it is often underdiagnosed. People within the low range of "normal" T3 and T4 levels are told they're fine, but they might have Hashimoto's thyroiditis, the most common autoimmune condition seen in our clinics.

When thyroid levels are too high, thyroid cancers need to be ruled out. The good news is that this is a rare reason for elevated thyroid levels, but it is one we do not dare miss, so we always check. Far more often the trigger for high thyroid hormone levels is an autoimmune disease, the aforementioned Hashimoto's thyroiditis, in which your body makes antibodies that attack your thyroid. The inflammation from the attack triggers the release of too much thyroid hormone. Medications can damp down this reaction, so it is a manageable issue.

The natural question is: What is enough? As people age, their thyroid hormone levels tend to fall. They become tired, fuzzy-brained, have low energy, feel cold, and gain weight easily. There's no need to accept age-related thyroid levels. With medical guidance, they can return to the levels they had when they were young, lean, and energetic.

Hormone Recap

As we age, all of our hormone levels decline. There's a solution to Mother Nature's unkind plans for your brain and body—replenishment of those hormones your doctors might not think are still vitally important for your longevity. Testosterone and estrogen (for men and women) top that list. Then factor in the likelihood of you having developed some insulin resistance, and every aspect of your health can suffer.

Once you've read this chapter, discuss any issues you have about your hormones with your PCP, an endocrinologist, or, best of all, a longevity doctor. If you start taking hormone supplements, it may take a while to adjust them to effective levels. Get tested at least every three months. There's no other way to assess your progress and adjust your levels. See Chapter 4 for more information on testing.

Chapter 3
How Inflammation (and Fat) Reduce Longevity

You already know about Dr. Mixon's Rule #1: Anything strong enough to help is strong enough to hurt.

Inflammation falls into that category with a resounding thud. Or rather, it leaves an explosive crater in your body. If I had the power to wave my magic wand and change American's behaviors in one way, it would be to make us a lean nation so inflammation levels would drop and fade away. Just that one change would cut our healthcare expenses significantly and start to empty nursing homes, because our seniors would be living fun, productive lives, rather than dwindling away in warehouses for the aged.

Much of this book makes clear that there are two potent, opposing forces competing for dominance in your body. Fat, which cripples and kills you; and muscle, which heals and repairs your aging body. Strong muscles that get worked every day are anti-inflammatory, repairing damage and helping you to avoid cancer and degenerative diseases.

But here is the crucial point: If you are sedentary most of the time and have a bulging belly rather than a flat tummy, that's a sign that there are big problems with your blood sugar, including some degree of insulin resistance. The more fat you have, the more inflammation you have.

In other words, a fat-dominated, sedentary immune response is pro-inflammatory. Your metabolism has shifted toward fat rather than muscle production. Your immune system is producing excess inflammatory products that will predispose you toward dementia, heart attacks, strokes, joint degeneration, and diabetes.

If that sounds scary, well, it should be. It *is* terrifying. You need to know what inflammation is and what it does to you so you can fight back and regain your health.

I have said this already, but it bears repeating: People who do not understand the incredible damage done to us by fat sometimes accuse me of "fat shaming" because I have found the need to use the word *fat* bluntly and make an issue of it. As a result, I have been accused of not liking fat folks. That could not be more wrong. I will continue to emphasize that what I dislike is not the fat people, but rather what fat does to good people. I am a physician. I dislike disease and disability. *Excess fat is the enemy of good health!* There is no other way to make you understand that if you have too much fat in your body, you are guaranteed to have chronic inflammation, and that chronic inflammation is going to cripple and kill you.

Inflammation Is All-Natural, But That Doesn't Mean It's Always Good

All inflammation is a natural process and a function of our immune system's response. There are two types of inflammation—acute and chronic.

Acute Inflammation

The acute inflammatory reaction is pro-health and triggers much of the healing process after an injury. If you break a bone or cut your finger, the inflammatory reaction sends out cytokines to attract help. As the blood supply to the injured area increases, the vessels dilate, and the platelets rush in to plug up any damaged vessels and stop any bleeding. Those platelets release nine different growth factors to trigger repair of the damaged tissue. In addition, macrophages arrive to see if there are any foreign bodies, such as bacteria or viruses, to get rid of. The macrophages start engulfing any damage, and any dead and non-viable tissue, to clean up the trauma so there's room for healing. As the healing process proceeds, the inflammatory process fades.

Chronic Inflammation

You *do* want the minor internal inflammation triggered from exercise. Whenever you work your muscles, ligaments, tendons, and joints, the micro-trauma to the tissues cause the growth, healing, and repair of the muscles. So minor inflammation is essential, as long as it's localized to where you want it. You don't want inflammation in your brain!

You *don't* want internal inflammation that becomes chronic and is responsible for destruction and progressive, painful degeneration. Any kind of damage that your body can't fix—a leaky gut, perhaps, where proteins pass through your intestinal tract to places they shouldn't go—causes destructive systemic inflammation with resulting harm to virtually every organ system, from head to toe. Another example is an arthritic hip that accelerates the degenerative process into the coronary arteries and raise your risk of heart attack, stroke, and premature death. Yes, you read that right. Arthritis, bursitis, or inflammatory joint disease raises your risk of cardiovascular injury or death. The inflammatory cytokines produced *anywhere* in your body circulate to *everywhere* in your body and increase damage to *all* of your body.

A primary cause of chronic internal inflammation is fat. It releases destructive cytokines, as well as increasing your senescent cell load, which lessens the amount of healthy tissue you can grow and heal and repair. This increases your risk of cell death, blood clots, and thrombosis. Your brain cells, heart, blood vessels, kidneys, joints, and even your retinas will die faster. Worst of all, your immune system will break down at an accelerated rate.

That inflammation is trying to destroy you.

Myths About Fat

1. **Myth:** Exercise is enough to offset a bad diet.

   Fact: In truth, most people cannot exercise enough to lose weight. Running a mile burns 100 calories for the average woman. An average smoothie is 700 calories. You do the math.

2. **Myth:** All fat is bad.

   Fact: We need structural fat in our joints, around our kidneys and bottoms of our feet. And we need fat to keep our brain healthy.

3. **Myth:** Eating fat makes you fat.

   Fact: Depends on how much you each. It is the total calories in vs. total calories burned that counts.

   We burn a certain amount of energy just staying alive. That is called our basal metabolic rate. Over and above that is the energy we burn through physical activity. If we eat more than we are burning, we store the excess as fat. If we eat less than we are burning, we burn body fat to make up the deficit. Since some foods are high calorie, containing a lot of energy in a small volume, we have to eat less of them than we would a low-calorie food to take in the same amount of energy. Fat is a very energy-dense food, so one way to decrease the amount of energy going into the system is to eat less fat.

4. **Myth:** You really don't need to add fat into your diet every day.

   Fact: Eating too much of anything, including fat, makes you fat. So the myth is only partly myth. But you can also get fat on fat-free foods, which often substitute sugar for fat. That is a losing bet, since sugar is high energy and triggers some pathological responses in our bodies that we do not want to encourage. It is almost impossible to eat a meal without some fat. Even vegetables contain fats/oils. So, there is no need to purposely add fat. If you are eating enough to maintain your body mass, you are getting fats.

5. **Myth:** Low-fat or fat-free products are healthier.

   Fact: Not true. The fat is very often replaced with sugar.

6. **Myth:** Saturated fats are *always* bad for you.

   Fact: Saturated fats like butter or shortening tend to be solid at room temperature. Yet they are also found in small amounts in unsaturated fats like olive oil. The 2020-2025 Dietary Guidelines for Americans state that you should get no more than 10 percent of your daily calories from saturated fat. So if you like butter, eating less than two tablespoons of it from all your food as your fat limit for the day is usually not cause for alarm.

7. **Myth:** You can target fat loss from specific areas of your body.

   Fact: Not with diets and exercise. But at our clinics, we have a machine that lets us reduce fat in specific areas using lasers focused a centimeter or two below the skin to heat fat enough to kill a significant amount and let us reshape your belly, chin, butt, upper arms, or thighs.

8. **Myth:** Eating fat will increase your risk of heart disease.

   Fact: This one is a question of genetics and other lifestyle issues. Sometimes yes, usually no.

9. **Myth:** You should not choose butter (saturated fat) over margarine (unsaturated fat).

   Fact: I like butter. It tastes delicious and does no medical harm in reasonable quantities. Omega-6 fats have their own metabolic functions that we need, but in our traditional Western diet we consume far more omega-6 fats than we need, and most people do not get nearly enough omega-3s in their diet. The imbalance results in significant inflammation and free radical formation. However, we live in a diverse society with a variety of ethnic backgrounds, and different cultures favor certain kinds of fats in their diets. My Chinese wife, for instance, does not cook omega-6 heavy meals, but our Russian neighbors eat very differently from us.

10. **Myth:** Omega-6 fats are bad for you.

    Fact: It's a question of how much omega-6 vs. omega-3 is in your diet. Most Americans have way too much omega-6 and not nearly enough omega-3 fats. At our clinic, we measure the 6/3 ratios so we can give you an informed answer.

The Link Between Inflammation and Fat: It's a Killer

When I went to medical school, we were taught that fat was an inactive storage tissue that just sat there. It was thought that the reason our knees went bad, or we had lower back pain was because we were carrying around extra weight, which put excess stress on our joints and vertebral bodies. The belief was that it was the extra weight that did the damage, and the cure was to put less stress on the back and joints. Rest and a less active lifestyle were thought to be the answer.

We were totally wrong! The reason we get back, knee, shoulder, and neck pain is because overweight people are people with inflammation. There is no such thing as fit and fat. You may be fat and strong, but that's not the same as fit. We need the minor localized trauma and mild inflammation that comes from exercise. We do not need the unending and destructive inflammation produced by excess body fat.

The Three Kinds of Fat

There are three kinds of fat. There are two that we want, but don't get to keep much of as we get older, and one we do *not* want that proliferates as we age.

The Two Fats We Want: Brown Fat and Structural Fats

Brown fat is a metabolically active tissue produced when we go outside without bundling up and/or exercise in a cold environment. Its high-calorie burn helps you lose white (bad) fat. Brown fat is common in swimmers, who work out in cool water, and distance runners who exercise in cold weather. They tend to be lean and eat more than the rest of us without getting round and soft. In addition to environment and lifestyle, genetics plays a significant role in deciding who does and doesn't get a full share of brown fat.

Structural fats are found in and around our joints, padding the impact surfaces like the bottom of our feet and giving us the full contours of a youthful face. This fat is found just below our skin and provides the soft, cherub-like faces and hands of young people. As we age, we tend to lose much of this tissue, in part because of the inflammatory effect of white fat you'll read about next. The structural fat in and around our joints cushions the impact of running, jumping, and climbing stairs. As these fade over time, feet hurt, joints start to ache, and skin, especially in our faces, sags and droops. Your hands and feet look bony, and veins and tendons stand out under thinning skin.

Your Brain Needs the Right Kind of Fat

Your brain is primarily made out of omega-3 fats, docosahexaenoic acid (DHA) and eicosapentaenoic acid (EPA). This likely explains why people who eat any kind of fatty fish like wild salmon, sardines, and mackerel at least twice a week have better long-term cognition than those who don't. When my wife was pregnant, I increased her omega-3 intake of fish oil significantly. Our daughter Ivory has taken fish oil supplements since she was a baby. My lean, healthy 11-year-old daughter has an IQ in excess of 145. How much of that is genetics and how much of it is the omegas is something we'll never know, but I do recommend an omega-3 supplements for overall brain health.

The One Fat We Do *Not* Want: White Fat

The third fat, which we cannot seem to get rid of easily, is *white fat*. It's actually a bit yellow in color. White fat is an extraordinarily destructive tissue. It produces over 80 peptides, hormones, and cytokines that trigger many, if not most, of the nasty things we experience with aging. Many of the cytokines produced by fat are immune-function products that prevent the immune system from finding and killing cells that are the unhealthy parts of you. As a result, white fat puts you at increased risk for virtually every infectious disease around, especially viruses like the flu and COVID-19.

How Obesity Leads to Disease and Illness

The following statistics are sobering. The risk of all of the following starts to rise as your percentage of body fat increases. We use the word *obesity* because it is defined as having a BMI (body mass index) of 30 or higher. The risk of disease is on a continuum; more fat equals more disease. As with all diseases and illnesses, prevention is far easier than treatment:

- Type 2 diabetes: Obese individuals are five to seven times more likely to develop type 2 diabetes than those who maintain a healthy weight (source: World Health Organization, 2021).
- Heart disease: Obese individuals are about twice as likely to develop heart disease than those who maintain a healthy weight (source: American Heart Association, 2021).
- Hypertension: Obese adults are more than two times as likely to have high blood pressure than those with a healthy weight (source: American College of Cardiology/American Heart Association, 2017).
- Stroke: Obese individuals are one-and-a-half to two times more likely to experience strokes than those with a healthy weight (source: American Stroke Association, 2021).

- Certain cancers: Obese individuals are one-and-a-half to two times more likely to develop certain types of cancer, such as breast, colon, and kidney cancers (source: National Cancer Institute, 2021).
- Osteoarthritis: Obese individuals are three to four times more likely to develop osteoarthritis than those with a healthy weight (source: Arthritis Foundation, 2021).
- Sleep apnea: Obese individuals are two to seven times more likely to develop sleep apnea than those with a healthy weight (source: American Sleep Apnea Association, 2021).
- Depression: Obese individuals are about one-and-a-half times more likely to experience depression than those with a healthy weight (source: National Institute of Mental Health, 2021).
- COVID: Having a body mass index of 30, the threshold for obesity, increases your risk of a serious or fatal COVID-19 reaction by 650 percent (source: CDC data on serious hospitalization from COVID, 2022).

About Visceral Fat

Visceral white fat in the abdominal area is the most voracious killer in America. Yes, we should be worried about toxic plastics and climate change, but fat is going to cripple you, then destroy your brain, and ultimately kill you. I don't know how to get this across to people other than by getting in their faces as much as possible.

Visceral fat is caused by insulin resistance. Whenever you eat or drink, the calories you ingest inform your body about how much energy is arriving. As you read in Chapter 2, if the amount of energy coming into your cells is more than the cells can burn in that particular time period, then the excess has to be stored. As fat. Thanks to Mother Nature, back in our cave-dwelling days, the fat we packed on for the winter was not supposed to stay there forever, or even for a year or two. It was burned off before the weather turned warm.

If only humans could be oil wells. Oil wells spout a flare of fire off the top of the rig, which is the excess gas that can't be trapped so it gets burned off on purpose rather than having methane (30 times more potent than carbon dioxide at raising temperature) go into the atmosphere. But we aren't oil rigs! Our bodies are designed to store excess food intake against a coming winter famine.

In women, fat is first stored on the thighs, then the buttocks, breasts, and finally, the belly. For men, fat storage starts on their bellies. This is due to the different estrogen receptors in our bodies. Women primarily have alpha estrogen receptors in the fat under the skin to make round, smooth female contours. Men primarily have beta estrogen receptors, so they get beer bellies first. Women lose many of their alpha estrogen receptors around menopause and develop a relative shift to beta receptors, which explains why older women start developing fat storage patterns closer to men's.

Is it harmful to have all that fat concentrated in one place? No. the harm is because the fat exists and it is a metabolically active tissue. How can you get rid of it? You've got to start somewhere and do something. Take the first step. If you do not start, you can never finish.

How to Reduce Visceral Fat

Step #1: Try to get rid of as much of that fat as you can by changing how much and what you eat. This means eating less food and putting less energy into the body than the body can burn in any given day.

Step #2: Reduce those senescent cells by moving more and creating muscle. (Or, let a clinic like ours reduce your senescent cell load with medications).

Step #3: Increase your growth factors as much as you can reasonably get them so that you can heal and repair; and raise your hormone levels so that your brain says, "Hey, I feel like moving today!" To the degree that you can shift your hormones with diet and lifestyle, do so. To get the best results, you will need to work with a longevity physician at a clinic like ours or an enlightened physician elsewhere. Everything and anything you can do to improve your hormone balance is a step in the right direction. That rise in anabolic hormone levels will help your muscles get firmer and stronger, which burns fat faster and makes it easier to lose weight over time.

Inflammation Damages Your Gut

Every human has more bacteria and viruses in their intestines than cells in the rest of their body put together. This is our incredibly complex gut microbiome. According to the National Institutes of Health, "There are 10 times the number of microbial cells in the human gut than in the whole human body, totaling roughly 100 trillion microbes representing as many as 5,000 different species and weighing approximately 2 kilograms." That's nearly 4.4 pounds of bugs!

The mixture of these bugs in your gut has an enormous impact on the state of your health. We can now identify certain bacteria that are linked to heart disease, dementia, and, of course, inflammatory processes. We can also identify other patterns of bacteria in our guts that are likely to help you be robust and thriving. As you might expect, active, vigorous, and healthy people have a very different microbiome than sedentary, inflamed, and unhealthy people.

When you're thinking about longevity, gut health should be high on your list.

The Type and Numbers of Bugs in Your Microbiome Will Help Determine How Much Inflammation You Have

We have a symbiotic relationship with these trillions of organisms living inside us. We provide nutrition for them and they process some of our vitamins and minerals so that we can metabolize them. We can't exist without them and they don't exist without us. We can destroy a healthy microbiome and an unhealthy microbiome can help to destroy us. It's a two-way street.

The different organisms in the microbiome kick out what are waste products to them but not to us, as we then absorb and use them as nutrients ourselves. With systemic inflammation, however, the microbiome sends things into the gut that change its ability to function properly.

Every cell in our body buds off tiny cytoplasmic buds called acellular vesicles. The larger ones are called exosomes. Both contain messenger RNA. In medical school, I was taught that these small vesicles were how our cells got rid of their garbage products once they were used up. It turned out that's not true. These vesicles are how every cell communicates with every other cell in your body. Healthy, robust cells are sending messages like, "Hey, I'm healthy, robust, and growing," while your sick cells are sending messages saying, "Oh, I'm in bad shape and things are not doing well here." I mention this because the bacteria in your microbiome are also budding off cellular vesicles and exosomes. They're also being absorbed from the gut into your bloodstream. This affects systemic inflammation by telling the rest of the body whether or not there are damaged tissues that need repair or destruction. The immune system responds appropriately to the messages it is given. Wrong message triggers the wrong response.

Since every person has a unique microbiome, how can you know which bacteria and viruses are beneficial? How do we make our bodies keep the good ones? While there's an amazing amount of research being done now, there is no diet that has profound effects on or will alter your microbiome. If you've ever taken antibiotics and had gut problems during and afterward, what killed the toxic bacteria infecting you also killed some of the much-needed good bacteria. Then as the bacterial load regrew, whichever bugs grew the fastest had a big impact on how you recovered.

Prebiotics, Probiotics, Postbiotics, and Your Gut

If your microbiome is not at its best and you want to fix it, there are three ways.

The first way is within your control. In order to survive, the bacteria in your microbiome need three things: the growth factors that come from our working muscles; the fat your body requires for energy; and fiber. They can digest fiber; humans can't. Eating lots of fiber-rich foods is a win-win for us all.

The second is a last resort for those who are seriously ill with gut problems. It's a fecal transplant, where stool is taken from a healthy donor and transplanted into the sick patient's GI tract. The hope is that the healthy bugs from the donor will colonize the ailing gut. Recently the FDA approved a pill containing a mix of stool bacteria that can be taken as a capsule, which is much easier to take than the previous, more complicated methods.

The third is by incorporating prebiotics, probiotics, and postbiotics into your daily diet.

Prebiotics

Prebiotic is a fancy word for fiber. The more fiber that gets into your gut, the more it will increase the bacteria you want in your microbiome, and the more it will preferentially increase the bacteria that can chew it up. The more different types of fiber you can consume, the more you're going to host a variety of bugs that thrive on variation. Eat more fermented foods; they contain a variety of yeasts and bacteria that will diversify your microbiome. Eat a wide variety of vegetables; don't just stick with carrots, lettuce, and cucumbers. (If you go to an Asian or Indian grocery store and pick up vegetables you're not used to eating, your gut will appreciate the new fiber coming in.) Yogurt, kefir, kimchi, miso, sauerkraut, and pickled vegetables are among the many foods that have healthy, living microbes that are good for your gut health.

Which brings me to the topic of dirt and your microbiome. Canned fruits and vegetables are sterile because the heat of the processing kills any bacteria. Fresh fruit and vegetables, however, are not sterile even though they may be washed at the farm, warehouse, and grocery store and in your home. There are still some hardy bacteria on them, and those bacteria came from the soil—those are the bacteria that you want to populate your gut. You don't need to wash these items repeatedly!

Humans are still animals. Back when we grew food in our own gardens, we ate some dirt with every meal. We are literally designed to survive thanks to a bit of dirt; most of the bacteria in our gut are common soil organisms. Our bodies are not meant to live in sterile environments. This explains why kids who live in homes that are constantly being cleaned and people who work in hermetically sealed buildings tend to have allergies and become sick with autoimmune disorders. Kids who grow up on farms and have their hands in dirt all the time are usually healthier than kids whose parents never open the windows. Kids who have dogs that go outside and roll in the grass and eat all kinds of stuff you don't want to know about, and then come in and lick the kid's face and the kid buries his face in the fur and inhales all of this dirt and crumbs are going to build a robust microbiome. Those kids have a much stronger microbiome than kids whose parents go to great lengths to protect them from dirt and germs.

In my military days, I developed a habit to help me stay alive in a dangerous environment. On those rare occasions when we soldiers were given fresh fruit, we gobbled down every scrap. If we left anything behind, it was a sign we'd been in the area and could be tracked and found. I had no idea that eating every bit of the fruit was helping my gut, too. Doing so became such an ingrained habit that I still eat the seeds and stems of my apples. You don't have to be that extreme, but eat the peels of your fruits and vegetables, and add fiber with supplementation if you need more. Your gut will thank you!

Probiotics

Probiotics are the beneficial bacteria found in fermented foods, such as sauerkraut, tempeh, miso, pickles, and yogurt. They are also sold in pill form as supplements.

Most of the supplemental probiotics are a variant of lactobacillus, the bacteria that gives the tang to yogurt, buttermilk, other dairy products.

It's not the kind of bacteria that is as good for our microbiome as the kind that grow in dirt. Furthermore, many of the probiotic supplements do not survive your stomach acids, making them a waste of your money. It's much better to eat fermented foods and the rinsed-off skins of fresh vegetables whenever you can. If you have a yard, growing some fresh vegetables is a step in the right direction.

Postbiotics

According to the National Institutes of Health, postbiotics are "substances derived after the microorganisms are no longer alive, or, in other words, inanimate, dead, or inactivated. The microbes comprising a postbiotic may be inanimate, intact cells, or may be structural fragments of microbes, such as cell walls." Think of postbiotics as the waste products created when the probiotic bacteria in your microbiome break down the fiber in the food you've eaten. They're also found in some fermented foods.

Why do you want them? Postbiotics promote the use of prebiotics. They're part of the microbiome's virtuous cycle. The more you have, the better your digestion, and the lower your risk of inflammation. As I've said before, it's all connected!

Think of it this way: Leaves fall off trees and decay on the ground, along with sticks branches, dead animals, and every other kind of organic matter. Plants use those decayed products as nutrients to grow new plants. The new plants are eaten by animals, and we eat both the plants and the animals. The same sort of process is going on in our guts. Old stuff dies and is consumed by new stuff, and the cycle of life spins on and on.

There are folks who wish to increase their postbiotic load for some reason. Personally, I have never considered it important since postbiotics are basically just how your body recycles cellular debris into new useful stuff. But if you do want to increase postbiotics, here is the way: Eat lots of high fiber, high residue fermented foods such as kimchee, buttermilk, yogurt, and soft cheeses.

Inflammation Increases Disease Risk

Life is dangerous. That's just the way it goes. I'm sure you know people who ate a healthy diet, worked out regularly, and had love and passion in their lives, yet died from cancer or another horrible disease at a young age. Last year, devastation arrived personally when a friend's healthy 11-year-old woke up to go to the bathroom and suffered a ruptured brain aneurysm and died. We are not immortal creatures, hence, as you know already, Rule #15: You can do everything right and things can still go to hell.

So, you do the best you can to minimize risk and cut down on everything that can possibly increase killer inflammation. While you can control lifestyle factors like food and exercise, you are unable to control genetics and cannot even know about the environmental factors that increase your risk for disease. Addressing those lifestyle factors becomes even more urgent and important.

Genetic Factors

You're stuck with whatever genes you were born with, but that doesn't mean you should just throw your hands up in despair if you have a family history of cancer, heart disease, or other conditions. Some genetic factors are influenced dramatically by lifestyle and environmental factors and can be minimized by proactive measures.

The genome is *propensity*. It's your risk of things happening, but it's not your destiny. The question is, are you going to live a lifestyle that will activate your destructive genes, or are you going to keep them suppressed and activate their alternatives?

For example, if you have the APO epsilon 4 gene, you are at a much higher risk for early heart disease and early onset dementia. If you eat the typical American diet and follow a sedentary lifestyle, there is a 50/50 chance that dementia will set in by age 60. By changing your diet and lifestyle and boosting your anabolic hormone load, you can reduce that statistic by 80 percent so you will only have a 10 percent risk instead. That's a huge difference.

You might also have genetic predispositions for a wide variety of cancers. If you have genes that are dominant, such as the BRCA 1 and 2, you have a 99 percent chance of triggering breast and/or ovarian cancer. (If so, the best chance of survival is prophylactic surgery to remove the breasts and/or ovaries prior to the cancer being triggered.) For most cancers, though, we have genes that can be turned on or off, a process called epigenetics. We may have a gene that puts us at risk, but it may or may not become active. Lifestyle and how much you suffer from chronic inflammation can make an enormous difference in whether or not you get the disease.

For example, women can lower the risk of breast cancer dramatically by boosting their anti-inflammatory cytokines through exercise, diet, and to some extent, hormonal supplementation. A previously sedentary woman who develops breast cancer can lower her risk of dying from the cancer by 25 percent by taking up a regular exercise program. If we had a drug that lowered deaths from breast cancer by 25 percent, people would spend vast amounts of money to buy it. Exercise is free. Why not use it?

Autoimmune conditions, when your body mistakenly attacks its own tissues, can be genetic or environmental and are on the rise in our ultra-clean societies. They are not on the rise in the developing world or in farming communities. When patients with common autoimmune disorders (such as eczema, psoriasis, thyroid disorders, or scleroderma) come to our clinics and we put them on our program, most improve drastically. We do not claim to cure anything. But reducing their inflammation and enhancing the nature of their immune response seems to improve their disease status. The top priority is to decrease the inflammatory markers in their systems to boost immune responses. This is done by helping them make changes to their lifestyle and dietary choices, as well as prescribing specific hormonal treatments.

Almost no one has just one autoimmune disease; you will usually find two, or more autoimmune manifestations in the same person. A healthy immune system protects us. Once that immune system goes awry, you're in trouble.

Environmental Factors

We live in a toxic world.

People tend to romanticize the time before the industrial revolution, but back then, life was short, nasty, and brutal. London fog was caused by wood and coal pollution. Raw sewage was dumped out the windows. Families breathed in toxins from chimney and fireplace smoke, especially in cold weather when the rooms were cold and the windows stayed shut. On balance, our current toxins are not as toxic as those of previous generations, which is one of the reasons we live so much longer than our ancestors. We seem to have a bit more control over not poisoning ourselves.

Just so you know, toxins, which in a sense induce biochemical trauma, damage us at the level of the basic chemical reactions we depend on for life. At low levels these toxins may not cause obvious harm—so their damage, being subtle and slowly progressive, is often missed until it is too late to effectively intervene. An acute poisoning is usually obvious. A slow, low-level poisoning from toxins in our environment is often, in fact, usually either missed or the symptoms misattributed to the wrong etiology. But a common result of most toxic exposures is increased chronic inflammation simply because inflammation is our body's go-to response to damage from any cause.

If you want to do everything you can to minimize factors in your life that unwittingly increase inflammation and other health issues, you need to become a savvy consumer to find out what's harmful. Avoid wall-to-wall carpeting, for instance, as it is full of chemicals like formaldehyde, which out-gasses over time. (Even wool carpets do, as the wool is full of lanolin that heats up from the pressure of being walked on as well as from the warmth in our comfortable rooms.) Hardwood floors are much less toxic, but colder and harder. That harder part is especially important if you have reached an age when you are prone to falling. Go for non-toxic carpeting or area rugs with non-skid pads. Life is balance and we need to make reasonable, not perfect, decisions.

Often the information about toxins in everyday products is not always easy to find. (The Environmental Working Group at ewg.org is an excellent source for information about toxic pesticides, herbicides, and chemicals.) Information shared by corporations is often distorted. Syngenta, the company that makes the pesticide Paraquat, has downplayed research that links its product to Parkinson's disease. Johnson & Johnson has long known that the talc in its baby powder was contaminated with asbestos. People paid for this with their lives. The corporations have paid in court, but that is no comfort to the loved ones of the people who died.

The Air You Breathe and the Water You Drink

The first few times I went to Chengdu, China, to visit Banding's family, the air was so filthy that I had no idea where the sun was. The sky was so grey that there were no shadows on the ground during daylight hours. We'd go back to the hotel at night and blow the black crud out of our noses that we breathed in all day. It has gotten a bit better over the years, but China is still a vast polluted mess. (That is a major reason that Western-made products are desired in China; we have a reputation for clean and safe manufacturing.)

In the Pacific Northwest where we live, the scenery is stunning, but we have among the highest levels of arsenic in our soil of anywhere in America. Rainwater and snow are potent solvents, and when they land on whatever dirt, rocks, and minerals they flow through, this leaches out the minerals and metals. If there are toxins like arsenic, cadmium, or uranium or any other substances in that dirt and rock, your water is going to pick it up and, over time, as it accumulates in your system, it can make you quite ill. A good starting point to deal with this problem is to install a water distiller or use a Brita-type pitcher with a filter in your home for drinking water.

In some areas of Nevada and Arizona, the number of heavy metals in the mineral-rich soil is legion, making the water taste metallic and undrinkable. Over time, you can develop heavy metal poisoning or sub-clinical toxicity. You may not show an overt illness, but you'll feel off-kilter with unexplained illnesses or a suppressed immune response. If lab tests show that your heavy metals levels are higher than they should be, an oral treatment called chelation can pull them out of your body. Never attempt this on your own, as the problem with chelation is that it pulls all the beneficial minerals like copper, zinc, magnesium, sodium, and calcium out of your body as well. That can be very dangerous, and is a treatment to be administered only by a doctor familiar with the process.

When the Rubber Hits the Road

Did you know that the closer you live to a highway, the higher your risks of cancer and dementia are? Thanks to the *road!*

When new asphalt is laid down, it's nice and smooth and your car zips right along, but as the years go by you'll start seeing gravel showing through the surface of the road. That nice smooth asphalt was pulverized into small pieces and sublimed into the air. In fact, millions of miles of asphalt highways are subliming into the air every minute of the day, so we're literally breathing in those highways. People often cover their faces when they're filling the gas tank because they don't want to breathe in the fumes, but breathing in the highway is much more dangerous. Over time, this can result in both liver damage and certain cancers. There are studies that show higher rates of serious illness and death in people who live near multiple highways. And yes, the vaporized rubber from tires, fumes from exhaust, and asbestos from brake wear do add to the toxic mix.

There are an enormous number of potential toxins, such as phthalates and glyphosate, that have been around for short periods of time, and we're still learning what their long-term effects on our health might be. Solar panels, for example, reduce dependence on transmitted power, but the panels themselves are comprised of toxic compounds like silicon and rare earth metals. When you need to dispose of those panels, where are they going to go? These toxins that you don't know about may not kill you, but they can affect your health.

Plastics and Packaging

Plastics are ubiquitous. A lot of them are toxic in ways that were missed by federal regulators. The regulators' job is to look for classic signs of poisoning when evaluating whether a product is safe to use in food and drink containers. Plastics pass these tests just fine. Here is the issue: Plasticizers, the chemicals used to make plastics soft and flexible, are endocrine disruptors. They affect how your body produces and metabolizes many of the hormones you need and use routinely. In this case, they have an estrogenic effect and are called xenoestrogens. The *xeno* means it is never found in any animal on earth—almost as though it came to us from a galaxy far, far away, as *Star Wars* fans would say. Our bodies simply have no genetic coding to prepare us to handle them, since none of our ancestors ever encountered them in the past.

In addition, when inhaled or ingested, plastics can cause inflammation by altering our immune modulators. They can also cause oxidative stress, heart disease, and cancers.

Skincare and Beauty Products

In medical school, I was taught that the skin was our main barrier against disease. Your skin is your interface *with* the world—not a barrier *against* the world. You better assume that some of what you put *on* your skin will end up going *inside* your body.

Think about everything you put on your skin that could cause inflammation. Read the ingredients on your shampoo or your moisturizer bottle. How many of the multi-syllabic chemicals can you pronounce or identify? Are these ingredients inert, a little toxic, or a lot toxic? Do they increase internal inflammation? There is so much we do not know about the toxicities of our skin creams, soaps, hair products, and moisturizers.

Once more, it's a matter of money. Everything in these products is on the open market. The testing for long-term toxicity is a very expensive and slow process, and no one has an incentive to spend that much money with no hope of making a profit from the investment. When we learn about an adverse effect, it almost always is as a mistake or an inadvertent observation. Oxybenzone, for instance, a common chemical used in sunscreen, was discovered to be an endocrine disruptor for estrogen and testosterone. It has been banned in Europe for years, yet is still available in the U.S. Except in Hawaii, where it was banned because it destroyed coral, not hormones.

Inflammation Causes Pain

Injuries create swelling and inflammation, which press on your nerves, which then send signals to your brain that you are in pain.

Pain is nature's way of saying, "Don't do that. Something is wrong." You're being warned that there's a problem. It could just be a stubbed toe, a pulled muscle, arthritis, or something as devastating as stage 4 cancer.

I've lived with chronic pain for almost all of my adult life, ever since I received my first gunshot and shrapnel wounds in 1966. My wounds don't hurt as much now, unless I do something really stupid and overwork my joints and muscles. I learned to compartmentalize the pain and not to let it prevent me from doing what I needed to do. (If you are successful at compartmentalizing, you know the pain is there, but you kind of shove it into a mental box and close the lid. I don't know how to explain that; it's just something I had to do to be productive. As you read in the Introduction, I'm held together with scar tissue and stubbornness.

Managing chronic pain wasn't easy. I'm so sensitive to narcotics that I can't take them because they make me nauseous and miserable. So, I was in pain from age 20 to 50, and was quasi-depressed much of the time. I powered on through because I refused to allow pain or fear to control my life. It was my job as a doctor to help people and I wasn't about to let some injuries from previous decades stop me. How could I still do that without aggravating even more of my pain? I learned to live with it. Yet as I got older, my injuries were acting up and I hurt more, so I became more sedentary. I had given up running; my back was hurting. My knees, ankles, hips, and elbows were causing constant pain. I used topical creams, cold packs, and heating pads, but it wasn't until I started supplementing my anabolic hormones at age 50 that my discomfort decreased significantly.

Young men have very high testosterone and DHEA levels. They are famous for doing outrageous things to themselves and think they are tough because it doesn't hurt. Once they start to age and their hormone levels drop to old man levels, suddenly everything starts to hurt. It's easy to be tough when nothing is painful, but not when everything hurts. Sex hormones, both testosterone and estrogens, decrease pain perception. As we age, pain increases because things are going wrong, our inflammation is sky high, and our hormones levels fall to the floor. It's not a good combination.

I don't recommend pain and suffering to anyone. There's no virtue in it. What's Rule #4? If it hurts, don't be a hero. If pain comes and goes and doesn't fit any particular pattern, get it checked out as soon as possible! If your doctor dismisses it yet the pain persists, get a second opinion.

Prescription Pain Alternatives

Sometimes you do need a strong painkiller. I have no objection to using them. I performed major surgeries for the first 20 years of my practice, and recuperation for my patients was often very painful. When a difficult birth left the mother in excruciating pain, she needed temporary narcotic pain relief. Heavy-duty painkillers come with side effects, but doctors know they need to balance short-term risks (those side effects) with long-term goals (healing and getting out of pain).

If you are prescribed an addictive painkiller, especially an opioid, take as little as possible for the shortest amount of time possible. Everyone has a different addiction threshold, but most of us have no idea where that is. If you surpass it, even when you're in terrible pain, you will become addicted to that medication.

This is why we're in crisis in this country with opioid abuse. Most of us don't understand the mechanisms of what prescription pain meds can do, so we're often under-medicated or over-medicated and can quickly become addicted. Fortunately, there are alternatives.

Non-Narcotic Over-the-Counter (OTC) Painkillers

Just because a painkiller is OTC and doesn't require a prescription doesn't mean it's safe to use. (Or if it's touted as "all natural." The hemlock that poisoned Socrates was an all-natural herbal tea. Cobra venom is all natural, too!) This means that when used at the recommended doses, the adverse effects are worth it as a trade-off for the benefits. The instructions will tell you this medication is for occasional use; certainly don't take it three times or four times a day for the rest of your life. But who reads the directions? Hardly anyone! This isn't smart. Aspirin is rough on the kidneys. Acetaminophen (Tylenol) is tough on the liver. Ibuprofen (Advil) can affect the heart. They might be inexpensive and easily available, but high doses can hurt or kill you.

The Safest and Most Effective Ways to Use OTC Painkillers

The safest and most effective ways to use OTC painkillers is with low doses of several different meds for an additive effect:

- The standard dose of aspirin is two tablets up to every six hours. The dose of Tylenol is the same, up to four times a day. Advil can be taken three to four times a day, depending on the strength of each pill.
- Take a dose of the aspirin. Two hours later, take a dose of the Tylenol. Two hours later, take a dose of the Advil. Two hours later, you're ready for the aspirin again.
- You now have three painkillers in your system, each at a low dose, so you aren't overstressing your kidneys, liver, or heart. The cumulative effect on your pain is going to be significant, and you probably won't need narcotics.

After I broke my left hip, I had three big screws holding it together. As years went by, the screws started unscrewing themselves and getting loose. I could feel them through my skin and they were causing just god-awful pain. I told my orthopedic surgeon to take the damn things out, as I'd been healed for 20 years and didn't need the screws anymore. He did. That left three large holes in my hip bone, but with my high levels of testosterone and estrogen I robustly replaced bone. It healed well in only a few months, and I didn't need any narcotics for the pain—just two aspirin, then two Tylenol two hours later, followed by two Advil two hours later until the worst of the pain subsided.

DMSO

When I lived in Idaho, every old rancher who spent all day on horseback would rub a liniment called DMSO on their shoulders, lower back, and knees, and swore it lessened their pain. DMSO is a horse liniment available at feed stores and online, and it's dirt cheap. But because it's so cheap, big pharma will never spend $200 million having the FDA approve it for your arthritic pain. I have used it occasionally. It makes your breath smell like garlic, likely due to a garlic compound in it. (Garlic is an anti-inflammatory.) If we're having trouble delivering hormones through a particular person's skin, our compounding pharmacist will add DMSO to the cream to make it more effective. It may be folk medicine—but it's folk medicine that many people have found effective.

Fish Oil

After finding out that 2,000 mg of a mixture of EPA (eicosatetraenoic acid) and DHA (docosahexaenoic acid) will often decrease the amount of pain people suffer from many common pain-producing conditions, such as arthritis or muscle strain, we often prescribe high doses of omega-3 fatty acids from fish oil as a dietary supplement in our practice. If you don't eat fish regularly or are allergic to it, there are vegetable and nut forms of omega-3 oils as well.

Acupuncture

In medical school, we were shown a film taken by one of the University of Utah doctors. He'd gone to China on a medical sabbatical and filmed an abdominal surgery done with the patient under acupuncture anesthesia. No medications were used. None of us could believe it as it followed no physiologic principles that we understood. When I became a country doctor, there were no acupuncturists around my small grain and cattle towns. As close as we got to needles was when a farmer stuck a pitchfork in his foot.

Joking aside, acupuncture has been part of traditional Chinese medicine for thousands of years and has become a successful treatment for pain relief in Western medicine as well, particularly for back and joint pain. Superfine needles are inserted into different points in the body to open blocked channels or meridians to allow your energy (chi) to flow better. Many people report that acupuncture is effective in treating migraines, joint pain, and some gastrointestinal problems. It is worth a try as it can't harm you and may well help you.

Testosterone and Estrogen

High levels of testosterone and estrogen affect the way your brain works. One of the ways testosterone does this is by decreasing pain perception as discussed above.

Estrogen is a potent anti-inflammatory, not just in your body but also in your brain. When levels improve, depression, as well as pain, can lessen so you can see the light at the end of the tunnel and not hurt as much.

If you have arthritis or another inflammatory process, a high-sensitivity complement reactive protein (CRP) test is a must. On average, the normal result is 1 to 3; with arthritis or inflammation, you may run from 15 to 25.

To treat this, look for any and every source of inflammation you can find and be aggressive in treating the underlying condition. Use the supplements we discuss in this book, eat less red meat, and increase your consumption of brightly colored vegetables and fruit. Move your body and look for doctors who offer cutting-edge longevity technology.

Cutting Edge Treatments to Reduce Pain and Inflammation

Senescent Cell Therapy

When the Mayo Clinic ran their first human study with senescent cells, measuring the chemical markers that senescent cells release in your body, that became the protocol I use (1000 mg of quercetin and 100 mg of dasatinib each day for three days, then four days off, followed by three days on, for a total of three weeks; that is a total of nine days in three weeks). The pro-inflammatory cytokines produced by the senescent cells went down dramatically—a 30 percent drop in only three days. This was a 70 percent decline in nine days of active therapy. This reduces inflammation while allowing muscles to heal, repair, and become stronger. When I knocked down my senescent cell load, my painful areas became less painful.

The prescription drug we use is approved as an anti-cancer treatment, so it does have significant side effects and some people cannot tolerate it. It goes without saying that this is a treatment that should only be done by a qualified physician experienced with this protocol. The patients in our clinics love the results.

The issue is we don't know how often to do the treatments, because it's so new. As testing continues, we hope to have better answers in the near future. The Mayo Clinic is currently running a long-term study treating dementia with senescent cell therapy. Think how many people and their families would be happy if it is proven successful.

Rapamycin

Rapamycin is a compound found in the soil on the Pacific Island of Rapa Nui, or Christmas Island. It's a potent antiviral, anti-fungal, and antibacterial agent that also alters immune response. It's FDA-approved for use in high doses after organ transplants to stave off potential rejection. But that's not what we're after—we don't want to suppress your immune response. What was discovered during animal testing is that rapamycin didn't harm the animals but extended the life span of every species it's been tried on. The higher the dose, the longer they lived. While it's the closest thing we have to the fountain of youth, it's a very expensive prescription drug and not without side effects. Back to Rule #1: Anything strong enough to help is strong enough to hurt.

I'm still experimenting with the dose and the form. It altered my bowel habits, so I'd be pooping three times a day, and all of a sudden I started urinating like I was 20 and not 76! That was great. But my blood tests were a mess. My blood sugar went into the pre-diabetic range. My usual total cholesterol went from 130 to 210. Since I cut down the dose, my labs have improved. But this drug is only about 11 years out from initial discovery, and its use in longevity medicine is far younger than that. We will be learning about the good and bad effects of this medication for years to come. One side effect is interesting and enticing. People using it often find that their grey hair is getting darker and thinning hair is getting thicker. Our compounding pharmacist is now producing a solution to be applied to men and women's hair. It's an experiment, but I have many patients who want try it.

The results are impressive enough that virtually every serious researcher in the longevity field is using it for themselves. I guess that says something! Adverse effects aside, it makes me feel wonderfully euphoric. After a lot more testing, let's hope this medication will become an option for many people in the future.

Inflammation Recap

Humans are genetically programmed to pack on fat. It's totally to be expected if those pounds have crept on over time, especially in your belly area. But this visceral fat is particularly harmful as it leads to the chronic inflammation that will damage your gut, leave you in pain, and cause a wide range of potentially lethal diseases. What to do? Number one: Don't give up. Number two: In addition to the pain-relieving strategies you just read about, every chapter in Parts II and III will give you the information you need to reduce inflammation while improving longevity.

Chapter 4

The Testing You Need—And Probably Don't Get

When I was in medical school, lab testing was basic. We checked blood counts, liver enzymes, blood sugar, and clotting times. We were looking for overt disease. When we didn't find a pathological indicator, we assumed the patient was healthy. On the other hand, in our modern longevity practice, we understand that robust good health doesn't mean there is no overt disease. Today, our goal is to see the absolute best level of function that any given human is possible of enjoying.

Fortunately, testing options have changed for the better, but the need for them is still the same. When you want to slow or reverse the process of aging, one of the best things you can do is get a comprehensive, multifactorial battery of tests that will address as many of your age-related deficiencies as possible. So in this chapter, I'm going to tell you about the essential testing you need to achieve for lifelong health and to be stronger, faster, leaner, smarter, and sexier. Without it, you risk it all—especially since everyone ages at a different rate, so it makes sense that you'll need personally tailored interventions based on your results.

If you are a patient in our longevity clinic, you will receive specific and ongoing testing. We measure hormones, inflammatory markers, insulin levels, homocysteine, IGF-1, and a host of age-related and functional markers at least every three months. Sometimes we test every two weeks for people with specific issues that need regular monitoring. We can do this because we have our own lab, which brings the costs way down; something that usually isn't feasible in a traditional medical clinic or doctor's office. Use this chapter as a guide for the testing you want your primary care provider (PCP) to do at your annual physical, and more frequently if you see specialists for any specific health issues.

Understanding the Difference Between Healthy and Normal Testing Levels

As you learned already, "normal" and "optimal" aren't the same thing. "Healthy" and "normal" are not the same thing when you get your test results, either. You can be deemed "healthy" by your doctor because your test results are "normal." But if you don't feel well, and you're putting on weight and feel your energy diminishing a little bit more every month or year, you may well be "normal," but I don't consider you to be healthy.

The problem with medical testing is that it's age-normed. The normal values and ranges of results for your primary care doctor's tests are calibrated to what is typically found in a person of a given age. For example, a woman who is in her mid-20s should have a testosterone level of 80 ng/dl. By the time she hits menopause, her "normal" level will be about 10 ng/dl. While this number is "normal," it doesn't mean she's "healthy" or able to reach optimal health at 60. Her lower testosterone, estradiol, progesterone, thyroid, and pregnenolone values mean she will be slower and heavier and have a lower libido than when she was in her youth. She will not tolerate stress as well and will probably develop some symptoms of depression.

In other words, lower and lower numbers become the "normal" as we get older. And as our levels decline, so do our levels of functioning. That's the basis for Rule #5: Just because it's normal doesn't mean it's good. Instead, you want to go for the *optimal* range for your age.

We draw these arbitrary lines in medicine and go by the statistical norm. Here's how it's calculated: Normal is everything within two standard deviations (the average amount of variability) of the mean. So we start by finding the total range of values for men and women in a particular test. Then we find the statistical mean. From there we go two standard deviations out from that, above and below that mean value. Everything within two standard deviations above and two below the mean is defined as normal. That encompasses 95.6 percent of the human population. It's just a statistical curve.

This, however, doesn't measure how you feel. If you're in the bottom 2.2 percentile, your results are abnormally low; the top 2.2 percentile are abnormally high. When it comes to IQ, nobody minds being in the top 2.2, but when your thyroid, estrogen, testosterone, pregnenolone, or any other value is in the bottom 25 percent, you would be considered "normal" but not functioning at your absolute best level. For many tests, you want to stay out of that abnormal range on either end. I don't want you in the bottom third of human functioning, even if you may be fine in the bottom 2.2 percentile from a statistical standpoint. You can do better. I don't look that hard at the "normative values" because they vary widely.

Remember Rule #3: If You Don't Measure, You Don't Know

Here's the thing about testing. Due to cost and time concerns, you may have health insurance that won't cover quarterly visits for many kinds of tests, unless you have a serious illness or condition that warrants regular visits and labs. During your annual physical, tests are done and your doctor then looks at the results. Maybe you will be prescribed certain medications. You take them, and if you feel better, that's the end of that.

Let's say you need more estrogen. What amount should be prescribed in a pill or a patch? The amount you're getting in your bloodstream isn't what you swallowed or was absorbed through your skin by a patch because everyone absorbs and metabolizes medications at different rates. How will you know what your peak and your values are unless you're retested after a few weeks or few months? That's why at our clinic we measure again and again when you start taking any medications. How else would we know if they're working or not? Unless you have an adverse reaction, assumptions are made by PCPs that the treatment is just fine and dandy and you must be on your way to becoming healthy again.

If you are undergoing any kind of treatment for any kind of issue, the only way to know what progress you're making is with regular, multiple visits and follow-up tests that measure and assess.

Alex's Test Results Were "Normal," So Why Did He Feel So Crummy?

I recently had a series of conversations with Alex (not his real name) about his anabolic hormone levels. He is a young man, which to me is anyone under 50. He found that his drive and energy, both physical and emotional, were declining. He could still have sex, but the joy and enthusiasm he used to find in romantic passion had paled. He wasn't one of my patients, but he knew of my work and asked me to consult with his physician. His doctor ran some basic hormone tests and concluded that Alex's testosterone level was perfectly normal for his age. That phrase, *for his age*, was the giveaway that there was a problem.

I suggested to my colleague that some additional testing beyond testosterone was indicated. Alex's thyroid function was considered normal, but it was in the bottom fourth of the normal range. His testosterone was normal, but in the bottom 20 percent of the normal range. His DHEA and pregnenolone were also low normal. His homocysteine was in the upper 20 percent of normal, indicating his production of nitric oxide to dilate his blood vessels was poor.

I made a few suggestions. We raised Alex's testosterone to the mid-range of normal for a 25-year-old, which put him in the top 20 percent for his age. We added enough levothyroxine to boost his thyroid function to a more robust level within the normal range. We added pregnenolone and DHEA to get those values into the upper range of normal, and a big boost in B vitamins to lower his homocysteine so his production of nitric oxide could rise. Three months later, Alex sent me a grateful email claiming that he has not felt so good since he was 19! His physician has since consulted me on several other problematic cases. I am always happy to help out.

Prep Before the Tests

One of the most helpful things you can do for your health is to keep track of your numbers so you can see what's changing or not over the years. Electronic records have helped enormously as they store your information from prior appointments for easy access. If your PCP doesn't provide information online, ask for print-outs of all your blood work and other tests every time they're available and keep them in a file. The more you know about your health, the better.

Three things that are very important:

- Bring copies of your medical records to your appointment if they aren't in the physician's system.
- Write down every medication and/or supplement you take, even if it's just a multivitamin. Even better, bring in the bottles. Anything that alters your body's metabolism is something I consider a medication.
- Write down any concerns and questions and bring them with you. This might seem like overkill, but trust me, it is totally understandable to have a high level of anxiety before any appointment. Anxiety makes people nervous and forgetful. I can't tell you how many times patients in my country doctor practice got up to leave after an exam, went to the door, and said, "Oh, Doc, by the way . . . " If I had other patients waiting, it became very difficult to spend another 20 minutes dealing with the issue the patient had been too rattled to remember.

The Testing You Need

Here are the basic assessments every adult needs when having a thorough physical exam.

Initial Assessment

Good doctors will start evaluating you the minute they enter the room. They'll look at your skin tone and color. Measure your weight and height.

Check your skin for any noticeable swelling or scars, and your hair (especially hair loss). They'll ask about any previous surgeries, whether it was a tonsillectomy when you were a kid or cosmetic surgery in your 60s, to assess if your health was affected. They will also assess how easily you get up and down from the exam chair, your gait, your posture, how strong your grip is when you shake hands, whether or not you have any tremors, and how energetic you seem to be. (People who don't feel well rarely radiate vitality.) They should ask about what you eat, if you take any supplements, and about your lifestyle. Do you drink alcohol or smoke cigarettes? If so, how much and how often? What kind of exercise, if any, do you do? Have you noticed anything out of the ordinary lately?

A basic annual wellness exam should include your height, weight, blood pressure, temperature, an EKG to show your heart function, and blood work. Along with way *more* blood work than is usually done! Women should have yearly pelvic and breast exams; those over 35 should have an annual mammogram; PAP smears should be done every three years until the age of 65. If a woman carries an HPV virus, she should not stop checking at 65. Men should have their PSA (prostate-specific antigen) checked for prostate function. Everyone should have a colonoscopy by 50. We are now finding late-stage colon cancers in men in their 30s, so I do the stool genetic screenings for young men. (If their insurance does not cover it due to their youth, it's still $300 well spent.) If you have good health insurance, hopefully it will cover all of these tests. But if your insurance does not cover it, do it anyway—you are worth it!

Body Composition

In our clinics we use a device called InBody, which assesses body composition and accurately measures muscle mass and fat. If your PCP doesn't have an InBody, there are other ways to assess muscle/fat, such as a nomogram based on skin-fold thickness.

Are You So Skinny-Fat That You Have Sarcopenia?

Our patients are often surprised when they see how much hidden fat is lurking in their bodies, especially visceral fat. The surprising ones are what we call the skinny-fats. These are people who are not overweight and they look fine. But when you measure them, they don't have as much muscle mass as they should; it's been replaced with infiltrated fat. This is called sarcopenia, a dangerous loss of muscle mass, strength, and function. When people with sarcopenia become too weak to take care of themselves, they often end up in a wheelchair or a nursing home and are at risk for premature death.

People as young as their mid-40s can be skinny-fat; they tend to be those who keep their weight down with their diet rather than with physical activity. They need more aggressive therapies, such as intense hormone therapy and senescent cell reduction, as soon as possible. They also need to start exercising more once their hormone levels improve; if they have such low hormone levels that it becomes hard to put on muscle, exercise will not be as effective at lessening sarcopenia.

Blood Tests

Blood tests can check a wide range of diseases and conditions. They determine how well your organs are functioning; assess your risk for diseases or autoimmune conditions; monitor any diseases you might already have; and show how well any medications are working.

Your PCP should be able to look at your blood test results, and then figure out a plan for your optimal health. In our clinics, we give our patients a notebook and they get their lab results as well as doctor's notes after every visit. If your PCP has online records, you should be able to access your test results as well as the doctor's notes through an online patient portal.

I wish I could say that a lot of PCPs will look at the tests we run in our clinics and know what to do with the results, but too often they don't. For example, they rarely test for progesterone levels in men or testosterone levels in older women. Homocysteine and inflammatory marker tests are all too rare.

This has become another problem in our medical system: For anything out of the ordinary that ails you, you are referred to specialists.

Orthopedic surgeons decide if you need surgery or not; for them it's an either/or. If your joints aren't great but you don't yet need surgery, they will tell you to take Advil and come back in a year. Your PCP will ask how you are, has the cough cleared up? It has? Good. See you next year. This is not optimal care.

Longevity medicine is a specialty. You would not ask your dermatologist to treat your heart disease or your child's pediatrician to help with your grandmother's osteoporosis. It is just as impractical to ask your PCP to care for your longevity concerns. Longevity doctors do tests and use interventions that are alien to the world most physicians inhabit—they are trained to treat diseases. We treat the perfectly normal but undesirable changes brought on by aging. Aging is *not* a disease!

See the next section for a comprehensive list of blood tests to request.

Vitamin and Mineral Levels

Without adequate micronutrients in the form of vitamins and minerals, humans don't live very long or very well. Sailors at sea used to die from scurvy due to the lack of foods with vitamin C. Think citrus fruits, berries, and tomatoes. Iron deficiency causes anemia and leads to a weakened immune system and lessened brain function. Thyroids that regulate metabolism can't function without iodine. Bones become soft without vitamin D. Every cell in your body needs vitamin B12 to function.

With the exception of vitamin D (which actually isn't a vitamin), our bodies don't make vitamins. But plants do, so the only way to get them is in our food. Blood tests measure these micronutrient levels. Our clinics use a specialized lab called NutrEval, where they take your blood cells and see how well they grow with and without different vitamins and minerals. The lab technicians look at 35 different vitamins, minerals, and cofactors. If your PCP doesn't use this lab (it's not available in every state), ask for everything listed on the following pages to be tested at your local lab. There are no standard levels of testing for vitamins and minerals because everyone has a different level of function.

Inflammation Levels

To look for systemic inflammation, we test our patients with a high sensitivity CRP (complement reactive protein) test every three months, along with homocysteine levels. Ask your doctor to do this as well. You need to know if this is due to excessive inflammation so you can take the steps to combat it.

Senescent Cell Level

Research is being conducted to try to establish a reliable blood test to indicate senescent cell load, but no widely recognized panel is currently available. The only reliable test requires a tissue biopsy. Biopsies of muscle, skin, fat, liver, etc., all show similar staining results to identify senescent cells. But every tissue releases a different mix of markers into the bloodstream, which makes finding a single marker for blood very confusing. To save the patient from this invasive procedure, we go by age, weight, coexisting diseases, and the patient's subjective response when undergoing treatment.

Basic Recommended Blood Testing

Complete Blood Count (CBC)

As I pointed out previously, there will always be variations in what's "normal," depending on age and gender. Discuss your test results with your PCP or specialists. Levels outside of the normal range will be marked L for low and H for high.

Type	Normal Range
Red blood cell	Adult men: 5–6 million cells/mcL Adult women: 4–5 million cells/mcL
White blood cell	Adult women: 4–5 million cells/mcL
Platelets	140,000–450,000 cells/mcL
Hemoglobin	Adult men: 14–17 gm/dL Adult women: 12–15 gm/dL
Hematocrit	Adult men: 41–50 percent Adult women: 36–44 percent
Mean corpuscular volume	0–95 femtoliter

Basic Metabolic Panel

Blood glucose
Fasting glucose
Insulin
Glucose-insulin interaction
Fructose sensitivity
Electrolytes
Salivary cortisol

Liver and Kidney Studies

BUN (blood, urea, nitrogen)
Creatinine
GFR (glomerular filtration rate)

Lipids/Cholesterol Panel

These are the basic lipid levels. If you have concerns about high cholesterol, perhaps a family history of heart disease, or you are overweight, ask for lipid particle sizes and lipid fractionation studies, as well as testing for products released from plaques. These subdivide your LDL and HDL into more detailed, multiple sub-fractions for a more comprehensive evaluation of your cardiovascular risk.

Total cholesterol
HDL cholesterol
LDL cholesterol
Triglycerides
Homocysteine

Hormones

Sex Hormones
Free testosterone
Total testosterone
Sex hormone binding globulin
Albumin
DHEA
Estradiol
Progesterone
Pregnenolone

Thyroid Hormones
The most common thyroid test is TSH, which stands for thyroid stimulating hormone. It is not truly a thyroid hormone; it is a hypothalamic hormone. The hypothalamus in your brain measures the thyroid in your blood. If it thinks you need more thyroid hormone, the TSH rises to stimulate the thyroid gland to make more. A low TSH means your thyroid hormone levels might be higher than needed; a low TSH means your thyroid hormone may be too high. This is the exact opposite of what most people think and is very important for you to understand!

The normal range for TSH is from 0.45 to 5.5. That is a wide range of normal. But as the TSH gets toward the upper range of "normal," it means that you have less and less actual thyroid hormone. Ideally, your TSH should be between 0.8 and 1.5, if possible.

TSH
Free T3
Free T4
Total T3 and total T4

Other
IGF (growth hormone)

Micronutrients

B Vitamins
Vitamin B1
Vitamin B2
Vitamin B3
Vitamin B6
Vitamin B12
Folate
Pantothenate
Biotin

Amino Acids and Metabolites
Asparagine
Carnitine
Choline
Glutamine
Inositol
Oleic acid
Serine

Other Vitamins and Minerals
Vitamin A
Vitamin D3
Vitamin K2

Calcium
Copper
Magnesium
Manganese
Zinc

Antioxidants
Vitamin C
Vitamin E
Alpha lipoic acid
Coenzyme Q10
Cysteine
Glutathione
Selenium

Inflammatory Markers

Complement reactive protein (CRP)

Other Blood Tests to Consider

These tests can be expensive and are often not covered by insurance. If you're worried about any of these issues, remember that your health is priceless and your longevity depends on it.

Plaque Markers in Your Arteries

If your cholesterol is high; if you're having symptoms of cardiovascular disease; if you have a family history of heart diseases; or if your blood pressure is unstable, a plaque marker test in addition to regular HDL/LDL cholesterol tests will show if you have early plaque, moderate plaque, or an unstable advanced plaque that puts you at high risk of a heart attack or stroke. These plaques put out chemicals, depending on how inflamed they are, so their levels can be measured. We can also tell how much of these particles exist and how large or small they are.

The Grail Test for Cancer

This test looks at 50 different cancer markers. If you ever had cancer, this test is highly recommended since people who have had cancer are at higher risk for other cancers. Tumors excrete proteins into your bloodstream, and the grail test can find them long before you have any symptoms.

DNA Methylation Testing for Aging

This test measures how much age-related methylation damage has been done to your DNA. (Methylation of your DNA allows us to predict with good accuracy your risk of heart attacks, cancer, and dementia.) Companies like 23andMe can only assess the risk of certain diseases, while this test looks at age-related damage. We now know that if you get a certain amount of methylation, it can lead to heart attacks and strokes as well as cancer formations and cognitive decline. Since we know what the methylation rate is for each age, we can look at your methylation and see, for example, if a 62-year-old person might have done as much damage to their genome as the typical 59- or 79-year-old person—to check if they've been doing a good job of aging or if they're aging faster than they should. We can actually alter those results by changing their hormones and lifestyle.

If you find you're functioning 10 or 15 years under your chronologic age, hey, you're doing a great job. Don't change anything! But if you're aging faster than your chronologic age, consider repeating the tests in six months to a year to see if any changes in your diet, exercise program, and lifestyle have turned things around.

Testing Recap

When it comes to testing, there is an enormous difference between "healthy" (what you should be striving for) and "normal" (the range that might not accurately reflect the state of your health). Ask your doctor to request as many of the blood tests listed in this chapter as possible and have them repeated regularly so you can track any changes. Equally important, make sure your doctor does not use age-normed values. Values "normally" change with age. You want the mid-range normal of a 25- to 30-year-old, not the normal of a 75-year-old. This is the only way to know what is truly going on in your body, and you deserve to know the answers.

For information about self-testing for cardiovascular strength, muscle strength, balance, and endurance, see chapters 6 and 7.

Chapter 5

The Supplements and Medications You Need—And Probably Don't Take

When I was in medical school, there was just one course on nutrition. I clearly remember being told that taking vitamin and mineral supplements was a waste of time. Right? *Wrong!*

The correct term for supplements is *dietary* supplements. These are substances to supplement your diet because what you eat is deficient in them. Here's the catch: *Deficient* is a relative term. There is *de*ficient and there is *in*sufficient. *De*ficient is a level at which overt disease will be triggered; this rarely happens to Americans anymore. *In*sufficient means that you don't have enough vitamins and minerals for your body to function optimally. This explains why medical school curricula, back when I was a student and even now, lead us to believe that most people don't need supplements because they don't have a clinical *de*ficiency. Our professors missed the *in*sufficiency boat!

As a result, there is confusion and hostility about supplementation even though countless peer-reviewed and double-blind studies have proven the effectiveness of dozens and dozens of different supplements. It takes a lot of time, money, and research to vet non-FDA-approved substances and many medical practitioners are understandably too busy and too overwhelmed to read the latest science.

This happened to one of my patients. "I brought in my supplements to my PCP," she told me. "Just a multivitamin/mineral and extra vitamin D because I stay out of the sun. He glanced at the bottles and shrugged. 'These aren't going to harm you,' he said, 'but you don't really need them. You're just wasting your money.' Well, he hadn't even taken my blood yet, so how would he know if I needed anything or not?"

Assumptions like this shouldn't happen. Yes, if you eat a healthy diet, you probably don't need dietary supplements. But what's perfect for you is not going to be perfect for me or for anyone else! Keep in mind that the food we eat often contains far less nutritional punch than it did in previous generations, thanks to soil depletion and the use of pesticides, herbicides, and other contaminants. In addition, the basic American diet is not a healthy one, so having a "perfect" diet is next to impossible.

Let me explain why good supplements are useful for just about everyone.

Dietary Supplements, Medications, and the FDA

About FDA Approval and Off-Label Use

What FDA (Federal Drug Administration) approval of drugs actually means is simple. Approval doesn't make a value judgment that the substance is guaranteed to be effective for you, although it may be for some people. What it says is that the company that invented a particular medication is allowed to market it for the indication it was approved for. In other words, think of FDA approval as marketing approval, rather than it'll-cure-me approval. This is where "off-label use" comes in.

For example, the FDA approved Hytrin to help lower blood pressure. Over time doctors saw that it also relaxed smooth muscles in the prostatic urethra as well as in the atrial walls. Ninety percent of the doctors prescribing it starting using it for men with prostate enlargement, not for blood pressure. This is called off-label use. Botox was originally created to treat strabismus (crossed eyes). When it was discovered how well it smoothed glabellar lines between the eyes, it took off as a wrinkle-relaxer and now has many other uses—to treat migraines and bladder dysfunction, to name a few.

While off-label use is perfectly legal, the catch is that the drug can't be *marketed* to doctors or the public for anything other than its originally approved use. Insurance companies and Medicare tend to approve payment for drug's approved uses and deny payment for off-label uses until the drug goes generic, hence cheap. As with many things in life, you get the correct answer if you follow the money.

The FDA Does *Not* Approve Dietary Supplements

Dietary supplements are an entirely different category than over-the-counter (OTC) and prescription medications. The FDA *does not approve* dietary supplements for safety and effectiveness before they are sold. You will see this about usage on the packaging: "These statements have not been evaluated by the Food and Drug Administration. This product is not intended to diagnose, treat, cure, or prevent any disease."

In other words, there is *no* U.S. governmental regulation of dietary supplements as to their safety and effectiveness. *You have no idea what you are putting in your mouth*—where it's sourced, how it's made, if there are toxins in the mix, if the dose you're taking matches what's on the bottle, or if the claims about it are true. Your one safety factor is the statement of it being produced under good manufacturing practices (GMP). GMP requires that the supplement be tested for minimal amounts of heavy metals, pesticides, insect, or rodent contaminants. As to safety and effectiveness, the FDA's only input is to make sure that a supplement manufacturer is not secretly adding a prescription drug to the product to enhance its effect.

From my perspective, distinction between a supplement and a drug is artificial. If an OTC supplement alters the way your body functions in any way, I think of it as a drug whether the FDA says it is or not. The doctors in my clinics prescribe supplements just like they do prescription drugs. The only difference is you probably don't need a prescription to buy the supplements.

Any medication or supplement you take can cause incalculable harm and/or addiction, even those you think are perfectly "natural" and benign. That this has become a huge problem in this country is the understatement of the decade. According to data posted by the National Institute on Drug Abuse, overdose deaths from prescription opioids rose from 3,442 in 1999 to 16,706 in 2021. (Read more data at https://nida.nih.gov/research-topics/trends-statistics/overdose-death-rates.) That data doesn't include deaths from street drugs and OTC meds and supplements.

Consumer Reports periodically tests large numbers of OTC supplements. They found that there's frequently almost no correlation between what's on the label and what's in the bottle. The label might say that you get 500 mg of that product, yet there may be 200 or 900 mg—and *there's no way to know*. Since there are no federal or state guidelines whatsoever, the quality control on most supplements is abysmal. The amount of active ingredients in any given capsule is purely up to the manufacturer. Supplement scammers take advantage of this lack of regulation, so you could be taking contaminated sugar pills for all you know.

Much of the harm is due to a lack of knowledge about the good and bad effects of what any pills in any form can do. It's why Rule #1 is: Anything strong enough to help is strong enough to hurt. Do you check out all the information that comes with a new prescription or OTC meds? You know, those densely worded, incomprehensible inserts with type so tiny—really helpful for seniors!—you need a magnifying glass to read? Most people don't. This is where side effects and contraindications are listed, so be sure to read them.

Furthermore, it's not just supplements that have issues. The federal government permits a generic prescription drug to vary up to 20 percent from the standards in the branded name drug. So if your prescription is for 500 mg you might be actually getting 400 or 600 mg. Why is this allowed? Costs, of course; the profit margin is smaller. Did you know that 90 percent of the generic drugs sold in the US are made in China and India? They do the generics, while American manufacturers produce the branded medications.

That bothered me when I first started my clinic, because I knew that when I told my patients what supplements they needed, I would never really know what they were actually ingesting. That's one of the reasons I started my own supplement company. I didn't do so until I found a supplement manufacturer that accepted my terms: I would test every single batch they produced, and if the ingredients varied more than 5 percent from the label, it would be rejected. The doctors in my clinics prescribe supplements, just like we do prescription drugs. Our patients can be certain that they're taking what they truly need, and if they buy our supplements, they are assured that they're getting an accurate dose that will give them better results.

Don't Believe the Hype: Just Because It's OTC Doesn't Mean It's Safe

Word to the wise: Just because you can buy some medications and supplements over the counter doesn't mean they're safe to use. OTC pain relievers, for example, are either acetaminophen (Tylenol) or nonsteroidal anti-inflammatory drugs (NSAIDs) such as ibuprofen (Advil), naproxen, and aspirin. Acetaminophen is processed by your liver, and taking too much can damage it and even kill you. NSAIDs are processed by your kidneys, and taking too much can damage them and even kill you.

Rule #2 exists for a life-saving reason: The correct medication dose is one that's just enough to do the job. It's human nature to think that if one painkiller is going to work, then two will work doubly well, but this is just not true. You can unwittingly put yourself at risk for some very unpleasant side effects. In my decades of medical practice, I have admitted people to the ICU with liver failure from Tylenol overdoses, even though they swore they took only took two pills three or four times a day. They were also heavy drinkers with compromised liver function, and were unable to eliminate the drug as quickly as most people. I have also admitted people to the ICU with brain edema (swelling) due to drinking too much water, which washed out their serum sodium levels. Yes, even water can kill you when used in the wrong amount.

Use the sidebar on the next page to find sites where you can investigate medical claims for different supplements. Read *Consumer Reports*. Some of the information is behind a paywall, but the website has a lot of free and accurate information as well. There are reputable supplement manufacturers, but there are far more scammers who cut corners for profit. You might be paying the price with your health.

If your concerns about your flagging energy have been dismissed but you still feel blah, Dr. Google is there for you 24/7. In a flash, Dr. Google sends you to his partner Dr. Quack, with that enticing list of supplements promising to make you full of pep again. You'll sleep better! Burn fat overnight! Change your life! Don't fall for the hype!

Where to Get Legitimate Information About Supplements and Medications Online

Government Sites

Centers for Disease Control and Prevention (CDC)—cdc.gov
Drug Enforcement Administration (DEA)—dea.gov
Food and Drug Administration (FDA)—fda.gov
Medline Plus—medlineplus.gov
National Institute on Aging—nia.nih.gov
National Institute on Drug Abuse—nida.nih.gov
National Institutes of Health—nih.gov

Medical/Other Sites

Consumer Reports—consumerreports.org
Drugs.com
Environmental Working Group—ewg.org
Harvard Health—health.harvard.edu
Healthline—healthline.com
Mayo Clinic—mayoclinic.org
Medscape—medscape.com
WebMD—webmd.com

Please Do Not Self-Diagnose

How do you know which supplements you need? How can you know if the product works, contains the correct dose, isn't contaminated, or if some or all of the claims are just quackery? It's not easy. It's far easier to want to believe the claims and to mistake what you see in ads and on labels for reality. I employ both MDs and NDs (naturopathic doctors, who concentrate on whole-body and more holistic treatments) in my clinics. When I hire MDs, they need to be taught about supplements and lifestyle. When I hire NDs, they need to learn more about pharmacology. I find that having MD and ND physicians in the same clinic and teaching each other is useful and of benefit to our patients.

When we evaluate a new patient, we ask them to bring in all their supplements so we can see what they're taking. More often than not, people will come in with a shopping bag full of bottles. They're spending hundreds of dollars every month—more than the cost for a month of visits at our clinics!

Worse, when we go through their supplements, we often find duplicates; they're taking the same supplement in three different brands and three different products, getting a massive dose of one ingredient and not nearly enough of the ingredient they thought they really needed. If they've come in with 34 different supplements, they're likely to leave with that whittled down to a dozen or less once we identify the duplicates. They might not even need anywhere close to that dozen either, but they're often emotionally attached to their supplementation, even if it's bogus. That's where the placebo effect can make them feel better.

About the Placebo Effect

I look at placebo as a kind of symbolic magic that symbolizes something of known benefit to have an impact in the tangible, real world. The symbol can be a voodoo doll or a lock of someone's hair or a good luck charm; in medicine, it is an inert substance. During the testing process for new drugs, they have to be compared to something that will have absolutely no effect on the human body. During double-blind studies, half of the participants get the actual drug and half get the placebo. They look, smell, taste, and feel exactly the same. (When a study is double-blind, not even the researchers know who's received which one.) The placebo is the magical symbol of the drug.

And guess what? A placebo sometimes works. Belief is probably how magic works. You believe it; it happens. Whether for cancer, high blood pressure, or other conditions, some people improve when they only take the placebo. Researchers and doctors are always dumbfounded when this happens. They want to know why the patient improved when there was no medical reason for it. *Something* gets tapped into that alters physiology. Was it a chemical change in their body? An electrical field? Mother Nature deciding to be nice, for once? The power of prayer or meditation? I certainly don't know why it happens, except to say that I'm a scientist who believes in the science I read about in studies, yet I also recognize there is magic in the universe, even if my colleagues don't want to admit it. From a practical standpoint, when we do a study, we are trying to establish whether or not our medical intervention is statistically more effective than symbolic magic.

Believe me, if we could pinpoint why placebos work so well some of the time, we'd be able to cure a lot of diseases. If I knew the answers, I'd do everything I could to re-create them and to teach others about them. So when it does happen, I don't ignore or dismiss it. I accept that there is magic in the universe that I just don't understand. I'm happy when anyone feels better or is cured by any means.

If you're willing to spend money on supplements through self-diagnosis, it's far wiser to spend less money on blood tests that will tell you exactly where your insufficiencies are. That way you won't waste your money or cause potential harm to your body. Also, state laws vary. In Washington, for example, you don't need a prescription for blood work. There are also online sites that explain how you can use direct-to-consumer labs in some states. They provide a doctor's reference for testing without you needing to see that doctor, which can be helpful for those without insurance or with large co-pays.

Once you receive your test results from your doctor about any deficiencies, then *take only what's necessary*. Every supplement, even those from the most reputable company, has the potential for side effects. I have seen many patients develop intensely itchy rashes while taking ashwagandha, for example, although it's a beneficial herb for stress relief. I always warn people that this particular supplement has drawbacks before suggesting they use it. You never know how you're going to react to any supplement until you take it.

Basic Supplements for Daily Health

Choose the Best Formulation for Your Needs

Many vitamins and minerals come in different formulations to target specific needs. It's worth asking your doctor for advice. Take magnesium, for example. If you're constipated, magnesium citrate stays in the gut and pulls in a lot of water, which can relieve the issue, but you can't absorb a lot of it into your system because it's staying put. If you want magnesium to have more of an effect on your brain, take magnesium tartrate. Muscle spasms? Try magnesium malate.

This is where doing some online research can save you money and give you better results.

Daily Essentials Top Three

This list includes the micronutrients everyone needs, even if your diet is allegedly "perfect!"

Multi-Vitamins and Minerals

Vitamins: A, B complex, C, D3, E

Minerals: Calcium, copper, magnesium, manganese, selenium, zinc

Omega-3 Fatty Acids

Omega-3s are critical for brain health. As potent, diffuse anti-inflammatory compounds, they decrease inflammation everywhere in your body. They can relieve joint pain and stiffness. They may also lower your risk of heart disease. If you take enough, it will loosen your stool to reduce constipation. How much is too much is highly individualized.

Resveratrol

This potent antioxidant can improve cognition and slow the formation of senescent cells. (The levels found in red wine and grape juice are very low, so supplementation is needed.)

What About Vitamin D?

Vitamin D isn't actually a vitamin; it's a seco-steroid hormone. (By definition, your body can't make a vitamin; it needs to be ingested.) Exposure to the ultraviolet light of the sun is what triggers your body to produce vitamin D, which is an anti-cancer, pro-bone-growth, and pro healthy immune system substance.

There have been multiple studies done with school-age children showing that higher vitamin D levels lead to better cognitive performance. Adequate levels are needed to help your body absorb calcium for strong bones. This vitamin may also help your immune system and reduce depression and anxiety. Many people are vitamin D *in*sufficient, not *de*ficient. In the US, we rarely see rickets, a disease caused by deficient vitamin D levels, but we have insufficient vitamin D for optimal health.

Controversies about vitamin D center around safe amounts to take. Normal blood levels are anything below 13 ng/ml, but improvements in bone density and in immune responses have been found in those who take 60 to 70 ng/ml and cognitive improvement in children continues to go up to as high as 100. The toxic range is believed to be 110+ ng/ml. We often prescribe vitamin D as a supplement as it needs sunshine to be activated but too much exposure can lead to skin cancer and photo-aging damage to the skin. Most people who live in the rainy and cloudy Northwest have a range of 25 to 30. The target for most of our patients is at least 60.

If you don't have any blood disorders, vitamin K2 (which does not affect clotting like vitamin K does) helps improve your body's absorption of D3. Many quality supplements contain both.

You Might Also Need These Supplements

No one has to take all of these! Have comprehensive blood work done to see where you might have any specific needs, and discuss them with your doctor to avoid any complications or contraindications, especially if you are currently taking any OTC or prescription medications. This is especially important for diabetics. Follow the directions and never take more than the recommended amount. Some supplements such as probiotics require refrigeration. If you have trouble swallowing pills or capsules, see if a liquid formula is available.

Acetyl-L-Carnitine

A form of the amino acid L-carnitine, this supplement can improve heart health as well as reduce insulin resistance. This form of carnitine has also been shown to improve age-related cognitive function.

Alpha-Lipoic Acid

This supplement is good for neurologic and cardiovascular issues. Make sure you take it with food and eight ounces of water. The acid in alpha-lipoic acid can cause acid reflux so painful that people think they're having heart attacks.

Amino Acids: Glutamine, Homocysteine, NAC, L-Theanine

The building blocks of protein, supplemental amino acids can improve muscle strength. They can be helpful for those who don't eat enough protein.

Ashwagandha

Used for hundreds of years in Ayurvedic medicine in India, ashwagandha is primarily used for its calming activity and stress relief. It can also improve libido and concentration, and reduce blood sugar, inflammation, and joint pain. Just be wary of the potential side effects listed on page 128.

Astaxanthin

Another supplement for energy and strength, it contains the reddish-pink pigment (a carotenoid) found in salmon that allows them to extend vast amounts of energy swimming upstream and jumping up over waterfalls to find a place to spawn. A 2018 study done at the University of Washington found that seniors who took 10 mg a day for several months increased their strength and endurance.

Astralagus

Best-known for its anti-inflammatory properties, astralagus is a Chinese plant also used for heart health, to reduce complications of diabetes, and as an anti-viral.

Berberine

The OTC alternative to the prescription drug metformin, berberine can regulate blood sugar and reduce triglycerides and LDL cholesterol, making it a useful supplement for weight loss.

Chromium

Although a deficiency of the mineral chromium is rare in the U.S., taking a supplement can improve blood sugar control and reduce insulin resistance and LDL cholesterol levels. If you're already taking insulin and/or metformin, however, chromium can further lower blood sugar levels. Do not take it without consulting your doctor.

Citicoline

Citicoline is used to supplement cognitive function and to improve memory, concentration, and focus. Claims have been made that it's an alternative to the prescription drug Adderall, but I don't see that degree of improved alertness or concentration in patients.

Coenzyme Q10

Another powerful antioxidant, it can also slow the formation of senescent cells. Studies have shown that it has a similar effect as astaxanthin, but is less potent. Statins, used to lower cholesterol, consume CoQ10. If you are on a statin, make sure you use 200 mg or so of this supplement.

Curcumin

Curcumin is an anti-inflammatory that gives turmeric its distinct yellow hue. It is one of the four ingredients in my Relief Factor supplement. Curcumin has been extensively studied and found to be effective when treating pain, inflammation, and stiffness. Taking a supplement with added piperine (the active ingredient in black pepper) makes the curcumin easier to absorb. A 2009 study reported in the journal *Nutrition and Cancer* found that curcumin and resveratrol taken together inhibited the growth of colon cancer cells.

DHEA

DHEA can increase testosterone production, so it can be helpful for those with declining levels. It can also improve muscle strength while reducing visceral fat. Some studies have shown it may reduce depression and improve skin texture.

DIM

A phytonutrient found in cruciferous vegetables, DIM (diindolylmethane) helps with healthy estrogen metabolism. Eating vegetables rich in phytonutrients is good for your body, but a supplement is necessary to get enough to reach a therapeutic level.

Echinacea

The purple cornflower grown all over the US, echinacea is an immune booster. It's often used to treat colds and other upper respiratory infections. Over time, it can affect the liver, so do not take it without a doctor's permission, especially if you have any liver problems.

Ginkgo

Often prescribed in traditional Chinese medicine, ginkgo is known for its ability to improve circulation in the brain. It is used to improve short-term memory and concentration.

Green Coffee

The coffee that many people drink comes from roasted beans, which is why it's dark in color. Green coffee is a supplement made from raw, unroasted coffee beans and contains concentrated chlorogenic acid, which improves glucose metabolism while reducing insulin resistance. It is mostly used for weight loss and has an anti-aging effect, particularly with skin to improve texture and reduce new wrinkle formation.

Gymnema

Gymnema can improve insulin production while reducing blood sugar levels. According to the NIH, it also has "antioxidant, antibiotic, anti-inflammatory, antiviral, anticancer, and lipid-lowering activities." If you are diabetic, do not take it without consulting your doctor.

Passiflora Incarnata

The purple passionflower can increase dopamine and serotonin levels in the brain, while reducing cortisol, so it's used to treat anxiety and insomnia.

Phosphatidylserine

A supplement said to improve the normal effects of brain aging by improving focus and memory, it is also used to try to reduce symptoms of Alzheimer's disease.

Quercetin

A plant pigment found in various fruits and onions with antioxidant properties, it can help neutralize the damage done to tissues by free radicals and reduce the number of senescent cells formed.

Saw Palmetto Berry

Mostly used by men to promote prostate health, and it might reduce the risk of prostate cancer.

Longevity Medical Clinic Supplements

Back in 1998 when I started Longevity Medical Clinic, I did not want to sell supplements. I believed that physicians should not "sully" themselves with crass profit motives. Okay, I was naive to the max!

The fact is that medicine is a weird hybrid between business and a priestly calling. If we get too far out in either direction, we are in trouble. Too far to the priestly side and we go broke. Too far towards the business side and we lose focus on the healing arts. So I started out by simply giving my patients a list of what supplements I thought they needed and sent them on their way. Then I became aware of three issues. First, patients were often paying outrageous prices for the supplements. Second, the supplements they bought often included other ingredients that I did not actually want them to take. And, finally, I came to realize that there was a great deal of variation between the doses on the labels and what was actually in the bottles.

As a result, I went to a small supplement manufacturer and arranged to have my own products produced. I required that the ingredients be tested by an outside lab and that any variation between the actual product and the label of more than 5 percent was grounds to reject that batch. This ensured that patients would be getting precisely what I prescribed, but as a side effect, it kept me from providing the cheapest supplements on the market. When faced with a choice between cost and quality, quality had to win.

I have carried these supplements for my patients since 1999, and a few years ago I started allowing listeners to my Saturday radio show to buy them. Now, with this book and TV show, I am opening their sale up to the general public. For nonpatients over 50 who want to use the most common supplements needed for their age group, I formulated the Essentials. They are a good starting point. Although I strongly believe that having one of my physicians prescribe what you as an individual need as a part of your care is a better approach, not everyone is going to become one of our patients. The Essentials are made for them.

Note: From time to time you might see me suggesting a Factor product like the following four. Full disclosure: I own a controlling interest in the Relief Factor Company. The Relief Factor Company website also sells my Longevity Medical Clinic supplements. So you will see a fair bit of cross-marketing between Longevity Medical Clinic and Relief Factor products. The same doctor designed, produced, markets, and owns them all.

In addition to the Essentials, you can try:

- Go Factor: B vitamins and taurine for increased energy
- Relief Factor: for pain relief and to make your joints more flexible
- Z Factor: for better sleep
- Zen Factor: for its calming effects

Supplements Recap

Because the FDA does not approve the content or efficacy of OTC supplements, you have no way of knowing what's actually in each pill or tablet. Since medical insurance doesn't cover nonprescription medications or supplements, consumers go online to self-diagnose, which is often ineffective, expensive, and/or harmful. There are, however, many supplements that can greatly improve your health and longevity but you need to be a savvy consumer to ferret out the legit claims from the hype. Take the time you need to thoroughly research what might work for you—and be sure to buy any product from a reputable manufacturer that regularly tests its products. This is why my doctors at Longevity Medical Clinics prescribe supplements to their patients just as they would a prescription drug. This is an area in which our doctors are experts.

Part II

How to Age: Stronger, Faster, Leaner, Smarter, Sexier

Chapter 6
Stronger

When I decided I wanted to stop being Fat Jerry, I bought the cheapest treadmill I could find at Costco and set it up in my living room. My rule was when I came home from work, even if it was 9:30 p.m., and I was completely exhausted, and all I wanted to do was turn on the TV to watch the news, I had to be on the treadmill. All I could do at that point was walk slowly. I wasn't yet able to run at that girth, but hey, I was moving. It took about two months until I was able to speed up and jog and then slow back down to a walk. Then I jogged more and walked less and finally got to the point where I was jogging through the entire news show. After six months, I was running. I burned up that cheap treadmill because it couldn't tolerate my size at a run! I was steamed about the money, but kind of thrilled that I was becoming leaner and faster. I got a bigger, better treadmill and kept on running.

When you start to move or move faster than you do now, you'll be just as thrilled as I was with the results.

Why You Need to Move Your Body

According to the Centers for Disease Control and Prevention (CDC), "Regular physical activity is one of the most important things you can do for your health. Being physically active improves your brain health, helps manage weight, reduces the risk of disease, strengthens bones and muscles, and improves your ability to do everyday activities. Adults who sit less and do any amount of moderate-to-vigorous physical activity gain some health benefits. *Only a few lifestyle choices have as large an impact on your health as physical activity.* Everyone can experience the health benefits of physical activity—age, abilities, ethnicity, shape, or size do not matter."

I put the sentence above in italics for emphasis. Don't you want to help reduce depression and anxiety, improve cognition, and sleep better as well?

There are two important components to movement: cardiovascular strength and muscle strength via strength training. Details about how to start moving can be found on page 158.

Cardiovascular Strength

Cardiovascular training helps to maintain and improve various aspects of heart and lung function by raising your heart rate and increasing your breathing, so they work more efficiently. When you work out, you will be less likely to develop heart disease or have a stroke. You will have more energy because your muscle cells use the glucose you ate for fuel as you work out. Your endurance will be enhanced, and burning up those calories will help you lose weight and become more active. Because you will have more energy, not only will the blood flow increase to your brain, but you will also become energized. Many people think exercise is going to make them tired, but the opposite is true! You may get physically tired, but you will become mentally alert.

Cardiovascular training also has a less visible but medically important component: It alters and enhances your immune system so you become more resistant to infections as well as cancers. In fact, the latest studies reported by the National Institutes of Health state that a woman who has been newly diagnosed with breast cancer reduces her risk of death by up to a whopping 60 percent if she takes up a cardiovascular exercise program. (That immune response boost from exercise is *amazing!*) Since every cancer starts with a single mutated cell, breast cancer has typically been present for two to three years before it becomes large enough to find and diagnose. What that means is that women who have unknowingly had a cancer for two to three years can still improve their survival rate by up to 60 percent by exercising even with the disease. Think about how much better the protection would be if women started exercising before the cancer even started.

Strength Training for Your Muscles

If you want to add failure to your workout, try strength training!

The key word here is *failure*, but not in the way it's usually perceived. With strength training, the goal is to put your muscles into a state where they fail. Failure occurs during strength training when you can no longer do one more repetition. That failure is actually what strengthens the muscle tissue itself. If you add more weight, that particular muscle will fail faster. If you are trying to do the exercise faster, the muscle will fail faster because there's less time between each repetition for the muscle to regain oxygen and blood supply.

But, know that this good failure of muscle strengthening can lead to bad failure, which is pain. The goal of strength training is to work as much as you can reasonably can on any given day *without* pain.

Besides building muscle, there is a hidden benefit of strength training. Working muscle produces a hormone called BDNF, or brain-derived neurotrophic factor. Yes, this says brain derived, not muscle derived, but the name was given when the factor was discovered. It was discovered in brain tissue, hence the name—even though the largest producer of the hormone is working muscle. The more muscle you have and the more frequently and intensely the muscle works, the more BDNF you produce. BDNF is a trigger to grow, heal, and repair neurons in your brain and peripheral nervous system. Grow those muscles and make them work.

About Your Core

Your core is the central part of your body, which includes the pelvis, lower back, stomach, and their muscles. Strengthening your core muscles is an essential part of your strength training, especially because we put on visceral fat in the belly area as we age. If your core is strong and stable, your spine remains upright and can bear heavy loads. Not only does this reduce existing back pain, but it also allows you to be more physically active while improving your posture.

Core work used to be dreaded. Back in the day, we were told to do endless sit-ups or crunches with our legs stretched straight out in order to get a flat stomach. Not only does that not engage the core muscles, but it also strains our back and neck muscles. You don't need any equipment to strengthen your core. When it's done properly, the plank exercise is one of the most effective ways to build up your core muscles as well as your arms, hips, and balance.

For more about how strength training helps your joints, see the next chapter.

If It Hurts, Don't Be a Hero

That's Rule #4, and it's especially important the older you get.

A while back, I took a nasty fall when I was trying to put the code into my cellphone while walking. (Not recommended!) I tripped over a curb and landed on my right shoulder, causing partial tears of three ligaments. The pain was excruciating. At first, I couldn't raise my arm without it hurting badly. After a few weeks, a colleague took some stem cells out of my iliac crest at the top of my pelvis and injected them around those damaged ligaments. They quickly started healing and the pain slowly subsided.

Before this accident, I was doing bicep curls with 45-pound weights in each hand. After my accident, I had to go back to 2-pound weights and could raise my arm just a little bit. When that stopped hurting, I moved up to 5-pound weights, and then gradually to 7, 10, 12, 20, and finally back to 45. It took time. It was tough. But I knew that if I pushed it, I would have to go back down to 2-pound weights and start all over again.

Bottom line: Listen to your body. When there's pain, stop! If you ever feel a bit sore or have any pain the day after exercising, you did too much. Back off and slow down some more.

Many people, especially seniors and newbies to exercise, are afraid they're going to get injured. If you do injure yourself, pay attention because you heal much more slowly as you age. Why? Because you aren't producing as much testosterone or growth hormone to heal lean tissues and encourage new bone growth, or estradiol to prevent bone loss, as you once did. That's one of the reasons younger people with higher hormone levels heal better than older people with lower hormone levels.

In addition, when calcium, phosphate, and other minerals begin to leech out of your bones as you age, that leads to osteoporosis, making bones weak and more brittle. Weight-bearing cardiovascular exercise strengthens bones. As a bonus, it also helps with balance, which you'll read about in the next chapter.

Take Exercise Breaks Throughout the Day

Studies have shown that children and teens who had exercise breaks in the classroom learned better, focused better, and fidgeted less. Ditto for adults at work.

An excellent way to get and keep fit is to intersperse concentrated movement throughout the day. In my office, I keep several pairs of hand weights on the windowsill near my desk. When I'm sitting at my computer and I get brain fog, or just need to get up and move around for a minute, I do some lifts and curls until my heart rate goes up and my muscles start to feel it. Or, I get down on the floor behind my couch and do some push-ups. Almost every day, I go out and walk around the block a few times during working hours, even if it's raining. I usually see several of my staff members doing the same, because I encourage them to do so. When they get up and take a brisk 15-minute walk, this not only make them stronger, but also improves their brain power. We're all energized and refreshed to get back to work.

There are many easy ways to move your body more throughout the day:

- Park your car farther away from your destination so you must walk more.
- Take the stairs—up and down—whenever you're able.
- Do simple exercises when waiting for something. March in place at the sink or after you've punched the elevator button.

- If you're watching TV and commercials come on, get up and do something. Unroll your yoga mat and do a pose or two. Planks are great, as are any kind of abdominal, leg, or arm exercises. If you've got kids, ask them to work out with you. That's a win/win for everyone.

Bag the Comparisons, Please!

Scientists have generalized human body composition, or somatotypes, into three distinct types:

- Ectomorph—Lean, fine-boned; doesn't bulk up with muscle
- Mesomorph—Narrow shape; muscular and athletic
- Endomorph—Rounder shape, broader bones; more fat and muscle

For instance, no matter how hard ectomorphs do regular strength training, they will not bulk up as quickly as mesomorphs or endomorphs. An endomorph will tend to put on weight more easily than the others.

Even if you start a longevity regimen with a friend of the same gender and you do exactly the same things and eat exactly the same amounts of the same foods, your results will not be the same. Your body types, your metabolisms, and your hormones all affect your results. If a man and a woman perform identical exercise routines, the man will show results faster. That's because men who are lean don't have the fat under their skin that estrogen gives to women, making it easier for men to get muscle definition. Women have a thin insulating layer of fat under the top layer of skin over their entire bodies that keeps them warmer in cold weather and makes them soft and rounded, as opposed to men who tend to be more firm and angular. It's unusual for a woman to get a "six-pack," unless she's a hardcore bodybuilder or an exceptionally lean athlete.

The only comparisons you should make are with yourself. Keep monthly track of your progress.

It's human nature to wish you could do your workouts with the ease and strength of others you see exercising. One chin-up is an achievement for a large man because for me that's lifting about 200 pounds. My wife finds it more difficult. She's only lifting 105 pounds, but she is petite and has smaller biceps that produce less upper torso power compared to me. On the other hand, she can jump rope at a furious rate, for an *hour!* I can lift her with either hand, but I could no more catch up to her jumping rope than that tortoise could catch the hare.

Before You Start

The Equipment You Need

You don't have to spend a lot of money to exercise. Walking, jogging, and running are free. YouTube videos and other tutorials are free. Many local gyms and city-run facilities have low prices or waive fees for seniors or students. There are also monthly streaming subscription services with low fees and options for hundreds of different workouts that you can do at home at your preferred pace and with instructors you like.

These are the items you need for optimal workouts:

- Supportive exercise shoes. For walking and running, make sure your shoes fit properly and are well-padded. Replace them as soon as the soles are worn or they lose their spring when you walk.
- Hand weights. For most women, one set of weights from 1 to 10 pounds is enough. If you're traveling and don't have any weights handy, you can use full large water bottles or a heavy book, as long as you can keep a firm grip on them. For men, dumbbells should be heavy enough to make more than 12 repetitions of curls and overhead presses impossible. If you can do 12 reps, increase the weight.
- Exercise bands, preferably with handles for strength and flexibility training.
- A yoga mat for indoor exercises to provide cushioning and prevent you from slipping.
- A great playlist. Music is one of the best incentives to get you going and keep you going. Smartphones make it easy to create playlists of

your favorite songs, and you can play whatever you like to match the speed of your warm-up and more energetic movements. I remember when the Sony Walkman became available, but you had to make your own mixtapes for the cassette player. Be grateful for modern technology that gives you workout apps and downloadable music!

The Mindset You Need—Longevity Is a Lifestyle . . .

. . . and you won't achieve it if you make excuses to avoid moving your body.

Many people who come to our clinics have never exercised. They want to feel better, get stronger, and lose weight. We tell them that if they want success, there's no getting around the point that they have to put effort into the program. The more they put in, the more they'll get out of it. If they aren't willing to do the work, we tell them that we will work *with* them all the way through, but we can't do it for them. Without them doing it for themselves, they will fail.

I often deal with this problem with smart people who should know better. One patient who's been coming to the clinic for years writes us a check every month to stay in the program, but she only uses her hormone creams and that's it. She doesn't control her eating, she doesn't exercise, she doesn't lose any weight. I don't want to stop trying because I'm determined to help her, so I've had endless conversations with her, saying: "I'm just telling you that's why you're going to become disabled and die young: because you're 80 pounds overweight and diabetic. You're either going to try to survive, or you're going to let yourself slide downhill and die. Those are your choices."

I can assure you most people do not want to hear that. But she honestly does not care. I get a shrug and a flat, "Well, Dr. Mixon, I don't diet. I don't exercise. And I don't feel like changing."

Make appointments to exercise in your calendar. Tell yourself your workout sessions are nonnegotiable. Because they *are* nonnegotiable. Once you make exercise a habit as essential as a daily shower or meal, you won't want to miss those appointments. Many men are solitary enough creatures to do their workouts alone; on the other hand, two guys working out together tend to get competitive, and that is a plus for both of them. Some people also find it motivating to have a workout buddy. Invite a friend and do it together. When someone else is depending on you to meet them, you'll be less likely to disappoint them (and yourself) by cancelling.

The Joys of the Endorphin Rush

One point I often make with newbies is how good exercising will make them feel. Not only in their muscles, but also when they get what's called a runner's high, or endorphin rush. Endorphins are brain chemicals we produce to make us feel happy. They are often released during prolonged exercise—not a few minutes of a leisurely walk—and can be triggered when you reach the point where your muscles may be exhausted and you're ready to quit. Suddenly, there's this amazing rush of feeling inside you that is pure bliss—several of my patients refer to it as an "exercise orgasm." The fatigue instantly disappears, and you find you can keep going and going. I wish I could say that you'll get this rush every time you work out, but you won't. It's worth the effort to hope that today is one of those days.

I can give you all the advice in the world (or at least in this book!) that will improve your health and longevity, but it's up to you to take it. You are the only one who can make that commitment to do a certain amount of activity every day, every other day, or every third day—or whatever—to the best of your abilities. We all know that life (illness, work or family commitments, inclement weather, travel) can get in the way. Don't let those things stop you!

Is It Worth Getting a Personal Trainer?

I'm often asked if it's worth hiring a personal physical trainer. A good one will teach you how to use exercise equipment properly and make your workouts more effective and less likely to cause injury. A trainer will supervise your sessions and show you new exercises to help you get stronger. I've seen people in gyms doing strength training and it's a miracle they don't get hurt. They're working out ineffectively because they're not doing the exercises properly. A good trainer can teach you proper form to prevent injuries.

The problem I see with too many trainers is that they make foolish statements, such as the infamous "no pain, no gain." (I'd rename that "yes pain/are you kidding me because there's no gain whatsoever.") Go back again to Rule #4 unless you want to end up in the emergency room and be unable to work out for months.

I recommend finding a trainer who is close to your age, because many younger trainers have no idea what it's like to have an older body. Ask around for a trainer who's lived a while and is still working out with decades of experience in the fitness world. That's the trainer who'll understand why you need to start low and go slow.

Assess Your Fitness Level

If you exercise regularly, you don't need to do this, but if you're a sedentary senior, you will want to assess your fitness and strength levels. The levels you discover below are your starting points—what you will be comparing yourself to as you develop your capacity over time. Whether you do amazingly well or find out you have trouble with some or all of these tests, relax. These are markers only for where you are now. If you stay with the program, you'll be in a different place in a year, or two, or three.

And remember—if anything hurts or you are short of breath, stop immediately!

Test Your Cardiovascular Strength with the Walk Self-Test

This test helps estimate your cardiovascular fitness, as measured by maximal oxygen intake, which is an indicator of aerobic fitness.

- Be well rested. Wear comfortable shoes and clothing.
- Warm up before the test by walking comfortably for five minutes.
- Walk one mile as fast as possible, preferably on a track, treadmill, or other flat, level surface.
- Write down your walking time, ending heart rate, weight, and age, then enter the data in the Rockport Walk Test calculator (exrx.net/Calculators/Rockport) to determine your score.

Test Your Leg Strength with the Chair Stand Self-Test

- Place a hard-seat dining chair (roughly 18 inches high) without arms against a wall, so that the chair doesn't move. Sit in the middle of the seat with your feet shoulder-width apart, flat on the floor. Cross your arms at the wrists and hold them against your chest. But you may need to use your arms for balance to safely complete the test: If you can keep your hands next to your chest without losing your balance, do so.
- From a sitting position, stand up completely, then sit down completely. Repeat as often as possible within 30 seconds.
- Count the total number of complete chair stands (up and down is one stand) performed in 30 seconds.

The number of chair stands you should be able to do in 30 seconds:

Age	Men	Women
20–29 years	27–29	21–23
30–39	24–26	18–20
40–49	21–23	15–17
50–59	18–20	12–14
60–69	15–27	9–11
70–79	12–14	6–8
80+	9–11	3–5

Test Your Arm Strength with Push-Ups

A simple push-up is a good indicator of your arm and upper body strength. Men do them with their legs outstretched; women do them with a modified knee position. Keep your abdominal muscles engaged and your back straight. Do as many full-range push-ups in good form, without rest, as you can. Stop the test when you can't maintain good form on 2 consecutive reps or cannot continue.

The number of push-ups you should be able to do:

Age	Men	Women
15–19 years	18–22	12–17
20–29	17–21	10–14
30–39	12–16	8–12
40–49	10–12	5–10
50–59	7–9	4–6
60+	5–7	2–4

Test Your Ability to Balance with the Stork Stand Self-Test

- Stand barefoot and place your hands on your hips. Position the non-supporting foot against the inside the knee of your supporting leg.
- Hold this pose for 1 minute.
- For the test, go back to the original start position with one foot against the other knee and then raise your heel to balance on the ball of your foot. Start the timer, then see how long you can stand without losing your balance. (If you're having trouble managing the timing at the same time as the test, find a partner to assist you.)
- Record the best of three attempts.

Note: Stop timing if the non-supporting foot loses contact with your knee; if the supporting foot swivels or moves (hops) in any direction; if the heel of your supporting foot touches the floor; or if your hand(s) come off your hips.

The number of seconds you can stand in Stork Stand indicates how good your balance is at age 50.

Poor	Fair	Average	Above Average	Excellent
10 seconds	10–24	25–39	40–50	50

Slow and Steady for Maximum Improvement

Whatever your fitness level, your mantra is Rule #13: Start low, go slow. Here are my guidelines:

- On the first day of your new exercise program, you should feel guilty for not having done enough. The trick is to start off doing significantly less than your body can do the next day. How do you know? You don't feel like you've done enough. In fact, you should finish the first day embarrassed at how little you did!

- Push yourself a little more the next day.
- Push yourself a little more for the following four or five days.
- After a week or two, you should feel much more comfortable with your exercising as you are up to the level that your body can handle comfortably without strain or pain. This is when you've reached a point that you're going to have to work a little harder to finish your full workout, so the muscles, ligaments, and tendons have time to accommodate to the good kind of stress you're putting on them. You'll grow enough new tissue so you won't get injured.

Don't rush your progress or compare yourself to others. Enjoy the time you're spending on making yourself strong and fit.

One of the remarkable things we see in our clinics is that older women with osteopenia or even osteoporosis often see their bones become thicker and stronger when they are on our program. The combination of exercise, strength training, and youthful hormone levels can cause old bones to improve greatly. I've had several patients tell me stories about their primary care physicians who expressed confusion and surprise because their DEXA (dual energy x-ray absorptiometry) scans showed thicker and healthier bones instead of continued thinning and decline.

We can add muscle, reduce fat, thicken our bones, and improve our mental functions as we age. But we cannot do it without thinking outside the box to improve our longevity.

How Much Exercise Is Enough?

The Cardiovascular Exercise You Need for Longevity

My basic rule for cardiovascular exercise is simple: If you're not sweating, you're not exercising. You need to move to sweat. This tells me that you've kicked your metabolic rate up to the point that your body is becoming overheated and needs to perspire to cool off.

How quickly you start to sweat depends on your metabolism, what the weather is like if you're exercising outside (obviously, you'll sweat more quickly when it's hot out or you're wearing too many layers), and how much you weigh. Those who are overweight have a lot more body mass to surface area so they don't have as much surface room to cool their body. Their muscles overheat much faster than a lean person's does. They will start sweating at a much lower exercise rate; they've exercised enough that their muscles are generating so much heat that they have to sweat to cool off that heat. It still tells me that they're burning more calories because their bodies are working harder.

How long do you need to sweat for? Those beads of sweat on your face, neck, underarms, and other places indicate that you're reaching your marker. The length of time depends on what your goal is. If you're looking for cardiovascular improvement, you need to get your heart rate up significantly—in the upper third of the acceptable normal range for your age—and keep it at that elevated level for about 20 minutes. That will give you cardiovascular fitness. As you get older, your capacity decreases, but your need stays the same.

Step to It—About the 10,000 Steps Marker

A commonly used marker for cardiovascular fitness is to take 10,000 steps a day. Subsequent studies have found that you can increase your longevity significantly by doing fewer—7,500 steps a day. Bear in mind, however, that every increment above 7,500 increases your survival rate while decreasing the likelihood of you developing significant diseases, although there is a point of diminishing returns. In other words, if you get 70 percent of what you're shooting for at 7,500 steps, 10,000 steps might take you up to 85 percent, but the next 4,000 to 5,000 steps might take you only to 90 percent. The more steps you take, the smaller your increments of improvement. (That said, I did 23,000 steps yesterday and I felt great!)

If you're already in good shape, it may take a week or 10 days to get up to 7,500 steps. At some point, you're probably going to want to increase your speed from a walk up to a jog. Here's how to start:

- Walk for 3 minutes, then try to jog for 1 minute. Or try to jog for 30 seconds, then slow down and walk for 3 minutes. Then try to jog for 30 seconds again.

- At your next workout, increase the jogging time to 45 seconds. So it's jog for 45 seconds, walk for 3 minutes, jog for 45 seconds.
- At your next workout, increase the jogging time to 1 minute.
- At your next workout, increase the jogging time to 1½ minutes. Then up to 2 minutes.
- Even if you think you can jog for longer, increase your increments at this point only by a minute during each workout. Within a few weeks, you'll be pushing as hard as you reasonably can without getting sore.

You can add intensity to your walks by using your arms. Swing them up over your head or to the side as you're walking. Try to keep your arms pumping for at least several minutes.

Use an App to Measure Your Steps and Gait

How far is 10,000 steps? That depends on your gait. I'm 6 feet, 4 inches tall, and my long legs take long strides, so I can walk farther with my 10,000 steps than my wife, who is 5 feet, 4 inches, can. Most smartphone apps have a GPS counter that looks at how far you went and is more accurate than the steps alone. Some will even calibrate to your gait, which is ideal.

Tracking your progress is important. You have a built-in measurement on your smartphone that can time and tell you how many steps you've done. My app tells me how many steps I took and indicates my vertical distance changes, showing if I went up and down hills or stairs. Be sure your phone is on when you walk or work out.

Use your app to record your steps for at least the last 30 days. This is the only way to obtain accurate stats, unless you work out on a trail or track that has a given distance. Otherwise, you're going to think you're doing more or less than you should be doing. When you're out of shape, it's normal to think you're doing a lot more than you actually are because you'll tire easily at first. If so, you'll be more likely to use your point of fatigue as a reference, not your distance. As you increase your conditioning, you'll do more and more with less and less effort.

Moving on from Jogging to Running

We all know what walking means. At some point, you will be going too fast for a walk and your gait will change into a slow, somewhat lumbering, version of a run. For me, that happens at about 4.5 mph. From 4.5 to 6 mph I consider myself to be jogging; at 6 mph and above it's running. But that's me, not you! For you, a jog and a run may start a good bit slower.

The rule is: Do as much as you can, at the speed you can on any given day without pain. Remember, *without* pain is crucial. If something hurts, stop immediately. If you're injured, you won't enjoy exercising.

The Strength Training You Need for Longevity

Strength training should target your arms and upper shoulders, core muscles, glutes, and legs.

If you're just beginning strength training, start with one- or two-pound weights and do 10 or 12 repetitions without pain or strain.

Do the exercises at a modest pace and stop when you can't do one more rep. You don't have to do two and three reps or two and three sets. If you do eight curls and your muscles start screaming, you're done for the day. What's encouraging is that once you keep at it and build up more strength, then you can do a second set followed by a third and then work up to using heavier weights.

If you can get to a gym on a regular basis, start with just two or maybe three of the machines at very low weight. If you're unfamiliar with the machines, ask a member of the staff to show you how they work. Try some chest presses, chest pulls, and, maybe pull-downs on a bar. Use them over two or three weeks until you can increase the weight range, then add another machine. A few weeks later, add another machine. These initial workouts will take only a few minutes, if that, because you're only doing two or three machines and you're not doing a lot of reps. That's just fine.

I'll say it again: Start low, go slow! Listen to your body; if it hurts, lighten up and pace yourself.

Once you start to build up your strength, increase the number and types of machines/exercises, the number of reps, and the amount of weight. My personal goal is to do 12 repetitions of any given exercise and any given weight before I increase the amount of weight. After I increase the weight, I might only be able to do six or seven reps at the new weight. I work with that amount of weight until I can do 12 reps. Then I increase the amount of weight again. This pattern will give you strong, but not bulky, muscles with plenty of endurance. If you do want to "bulk up," do fewer reps with heavier weights that stress the muscle to failure. A man in his 40s or 50s who's finally gotten to the point where he can do a chin-up will be able to lift his body weight with his biceps. That's a good amount! For a man his age, even one chin-up is an accomplishment. The guy who can do three or so is in excellent shape; four and above is an unusual accomplishment for anyone over the age of 40.

For details on a weekly workout program, see the next section.

How My Patient Richard Tonelli Works Out—at 86!

Richard has been a patient for about 25 years. At 86, he is doing great! He is the sort of fellow who shows what can be done. His long list of joint surgeries should tell you that we did not make him young—time and gravity are doing their thing on him as they do on everyone—but at his age, he is living a life that many people decades younger would envy. Here's Richard on his exercise routine:

I've always been interested in having a healthy mind-and-body lifestyle. I researched the benefits of supplementation, good eating habits, and workout training, which was especially important since I was a commercial airline pilot. In the 1980s, my workout routine consisted of weight training two or three times a week and running three miles twice a week. When my wife Karen and I first heard Dr. Mixon on the radio, his statements resonated with us: "Normal is not good enough." And, "If you don't test, you don't know." And,

"I want you to have blood work of a 25- to 30-year-old." We've been coming to the Longevity Medical Clinic in Tacoma since the late 1990s, and often listen to the Saturday podcasts. When asked why we're in such good shape at our ages, we tell our friends and relatives about Dr. Mixon and his program.

I am 86 years old, weigh 145 pounds, have around 16 percent body fat, and my resting heart rate is below 50. My blood pressure is about 117/70. I've had neck fusion surgery, three back operations, a right hip replacement, partial replacement of both knees simultaneously, a redo of a full knee replacement on my left knee, and most recently a left hip replacement. One thing that aided my recoveries was to concentrate on strengthening the muscles around the joints that had already been replaced. This made doing the post-op physical therapy easier and helped get my body back to where it had been.

My workout routines are divided into three sessions that I call Push, Pull, and Legs. They usually last from 1 to 1½ hours. I do the Push and Pull routines at home and my Leg routine at a gym using the machines and the treadmill. If I have any joint pain, I do just a rep or two. If there's no relief, I eliminate that set for that day's workout. Muscle fatigue is okay but I watch my form. I start a set every 4 minutes for my first set of five reps:

- For the Push workout, I do bench curls, bench flies, and stand-up curls with dumbbells and hand weights.
- For the Pull workout, I installed a pull-up rack on my laundry room wall for pull-ups and positioned rubber exercise bands for lateral pull-downs. The bedroom doorknob is used for the seated rows and rotator cuff routines while I'm seated on a bench.
- For the Leg workout in the gym, I do a 10- to 30-minute warm-up at 3.2 mph on the treadmill set at 2.5 degrees. Then I do leg

presses, adductor and abductor, leg curls, leg kickbacks, and leg extensions on the weight machines. I constantly have to resist the urge to do much more. My best gauge about whether I've done too much shows up in the next day or so with muscle and joint discomfort.

My goal regarding my legs is to allow me mobility to do things I want to do: getting up and down from the floor, hiking for miles, climbing hills, and dancing. I have added personal trainers for yoga and stretching, both of which help with mobility. All of my hard work paid off when I recently took a trip to Quito, Ecuador, where the elevation is about 9,600 feet. When I checked my heart rate, it was 55 bpm and I didn't feel any effects of the altitude. After being there less than a day, we took a gondola to the top of a nearby mountain, which was 13,400 feet. This time I noticed that I had to breathe a little more often and my heart rate had increased to 75 bpm.

Putting It All Together—The Longevity Workout Program

These are my basic recommendations for optimal training and longevity. A well-rounded physical activity program helps you grow in strength and activity by including cardiovascular exercise, strength training, stretching/flexibility exercises, and balance exercise throughout the week. For details on the latter two, see the next chapter.

Dynamic Warm-Ups

A dynamic warm-up coordinates your muscles, tendons, ligaments, and joints, and even your nervous system. Warming up challenges your flexibility, mobility, strength, and stability, and is essential in reducing the risk of injury while enhancing subsequent performance. Do these before cardiovascular or strength training, at least two or three days each week. Try to do some stretches after a workout when your body is still warm to help release any tightness in your muscles. Never stretch to the point of pain. Your body should always feel good!

Cardiovascular Training

Do cardiovascular exercise of moderate intensity, such as brisk walking, for 20 to 45 minutes each day; or vigorous exercise, like running, for 15 to 30 minutes.

A rule of thumb is that one minute of vigorous activity provides the same health benefits as two minutes of moderate activity. Each cardiovascular workout session should consist of a warm-up period, exercising within your target heart rate zone, and an easier cool-down period. Check your pulse periodically to see if you are within your target zone. If you find a particular week's pattern tiring, repeat it before moving on to the next level. Start at a pace that's comfortable for you, gradually picking up speed until you're moving briskly. You should be breathing hard, but you should still be able to carry on a conversation. Each week, add about two minutes to your time.

Strength Training

Strength-train two or three days each week. Rotate between upper body, core, and lower body to give yourself variety, as well as to work out your full body through the course of a week. Leave 48 hours between strength training sessions for your body to recover. Start with just one set (a group of repetitions) of each exercise per session. Progress over the next few weeks to two or three sets. Rest for two to three minutes between sets, if needed.

Stretching/Flexibility Training

Stretching will help improve your joints' range of motion, increase fluidity in the joints and overall tissue health, and improve your ability to perform daily tasks. Do stretching/flexibility training at least two or three days each week for 10 to 20 minutes. For each exercise, 8 to 12 repetitions will improve strength and power; 10 to 15 repetitions will improve strength in those age 50 and up and just starting exercise; and 15 to 20 repetitions will improve muscular endurance. If you are doing fewer repetitions, use a higher tensile exercise band. If you are doing more repetitions, use a lower tensile exercise band.

Balance Training

Balance training helps improve your ability to stay in control of body movement, correct yourself if you lose your balance, and prevent falls. Work on your balance two or three days each week for at least 5 to 10 minutes—the more, the better.

The Supplements You Need for Strength

Refer to Chapter 5 for more details. Discuss the proper doses for your needs as well as any potential contraindications with your doctor before taking any new supplements.

Creatine This is the most effective supplement documented to increase lean body mass and exercise capacity. Both short-term and long-term creatine use increases growth hormone production and the strength and efficiency of your muscles. The downside of creatine is that it is unsafe for those with poor kidney function or disease. If you have any kidney issues, do not take it without permission from your doctor.

DHEA This supplement is a maybe for some people. Many people suggest DHEA as a testosterone booster. Since DHEA has the capacity to raise estrogen levels in addition to testosterone, I use it with only our clinic patients since we check their hormone levels every three months. I disapprove of using DHEA if you are not getting your hormone levels checked regularly.

Neoforte This contains omega-3s, ginkgo, and other ingredients that increase nitric oxide production, which helps dilate your blood vessels for more efficient blood flow to your muscles.

Chapter 7
Faster

I love to ski. It's all about going faster.

About 24 years ago, I was glacier skiing in Canada when I made a serious mistake. While zooming down the mountain like a bat out of hell, I twisted around to see if anyone was catching up. I instantly discovered that looking *up* the mountain while skiing *down* the mountain is not a smart thing to do. (Living proof that you don't have to be smart to be a doctor!)

Anyway, I hit the ice going fast and sheared the ball at the top of my femur right off the bone, which is called a subcapital femoral neck fracture. I was airlifted to Vancouver and had surgery on my hip that night. The injury interrupted the blood supply so the part of the ball that fits into the hip socket died, leaving an irregular surface to erode over time. As you might expect, it was incredibly painful and triggered some arthritic changes. Since I didn't want a hip replacement, I discussed alternatives with a buddy of mine who's a pain management specialist. He took stem cells out of my hip bone marrow and PRP (platelet-rich plasma) out of my arm and injected both into my painful hip. Six weeks later, I had another set of PRP injections that got rid of about 80 percent of my arthritic pain. Six months after that, he repeated the initial procedure, and my hip has been pain free ever since.

The moral of this story? Think about what can speed you up—and that means thinking about your metabolism, because the more energy you have, the faster you can go. Also think about your joints, your flexibility, and your balance, which will make you go faster as well.

And never look up the mountain when skiing down!

Your Metabolism and Energy Needs

Most people have no concept of what their metabolic needs are, which can lead to many of the weight gain and food issues you'll read about in the next chapter. But first, let's go back to the basics of calories and energy.

Understanding Caloric/Metabolic Needs

What is a calorie?

A calorie is defined as a unit of energy equivalent to the heat energy needed to raise the temperature of one gram of water by one degree Celsius. When it comes to food, a calorie is used to measure its energy content.

Every person has different daily caloric needs to keep their bodies working. These needs are based on height, weight, gender, muscle mass, previous illnesses or medical conditions (such as thyroid dysregulation, which can speed up or slow down your metabolism), and age. Many of these factors are genetic, so they can't be altered. This explains why some people have naturally speedy metabolisms and can seemingly eat whatever they want without gaining weight, while others easily pack on pounds even when they eat the right amount of calories for their metabolic needs.

Measuring Your Own Caloric Needs

There are two ways to do this:

- Use a nomogram, which is a chart that has you input your weight, height, age, and typical daily activity level (low, moderate, or intense exercise). It will then give you a rough estimate of your caloric needs for the day. One of the best calorie nomograms can be found on this website:

https://www.mayoclinic.org/healthy-lifestyle/weight-loss/in-depth/calorie-calculator/itt-20402304. There are lots of other nomograms out there, but I think this is one of the better ones.

- See a doctor who has an InBody device. It can precisely measure your total weight and how much muscle and fat you have, and give you your metabolic caloric base needs for each day. I put them in all my clinics because tracking muscle and fat is critical for us. (It's a rather pricey machine, so you might need to call around to see if any local doctors have one.)

When I first saw the U.S. government's requirement that calorie counts had to be clearly listed on certain restaurant menus, I thought it was intrusive and unnecessary. I've changed my mind, because I hope that by reading the actual calorie numbers in food, people will modify their choices. If your metabolic needs are 1,600 calories/day and a smoothie has 600 calories, that one drink is more than one-third of your calorie allotment in the form of sugar and fat. It will taste delicious when you drink it, but do you want that to be one of your three daily meals? I doubt it.

How Many Calories Can You Burn with Exercise?

The more muscle and the less fat in a person's body, the more calories they will burn both at rest and during any activity. The more intense your workout, the more energy you'll keep on burning for longer periods once you finish your workout, as your metabolism will still be raised, and your body will be consuming more oxygen.

There are many online sites where you can enter your height, weight, and age and get an accurate number for what your calorie burn rate should be. On average, a 150-pound woman who walks one mile burns about 100 calories. If she takes a 30-minute walk twice a day, that's 200 calories burned. The greater the distance she walks, or if she is overweight, she will burn more calories. At my weight of around 200 pounds, I burn about 125 calories per mile.

It doesn't matter whether you walk, jog, or run, you will burn the same number of calories per *distance*, not by the amount of time. If you walk slowly, you don't get as many cardiovascular benefits, but if your goal is calorie burn, it's the same at any rate. If the average senior walks about 3 miles per hour (20-minute miles) and does a 30-minute walk twice a day, once in the morning and again in the evening, that's 200+ calories burned off each day, depending on their weight. That's a good start, if you complement that by being careful about how many calories you eat in that day.

Think about calories this way, too: If you cut down your daily food intake by 200 calories per day, that equals losing 20 pounds per year; a loss of 100 calories per day is 10 pounds per year. That's the simple metric. If you eat one extra 100-calorie slice of bread per day, you will gain 10 pounds per year. If you cut out that one slice of bread a day, you can lose 10 pounds a year. If you walk 30 minutes each day, you can lose 10 pounds a year. If you're not walking 30 minutes a day, you're setting yourself up to gain 10 pounds a year. The goal is to shift your balance by a certain number of calories per day, depending on how much you're trying to lose over the course of the next year.

To Move Faster, Strengthen Your Muscles and Joints

Do you hear your bones creaking when you get out of bed in the morning? Do your joints ache occasionally or all the time? Weight-bearing or moderate- or high-impact cardiovascular routines like running or jumping rope will strengthen bones but can stress joints—as runners who pound the pavement for years will attest. It's time to add strength training to your workout program as well as flexibility exercises.

The stronger your muscles, the safer your joints and the faster and more easily you will move.

Climb Every Mountain, Even the One in Your Home

An 80-year-old man came to the clinic with the goal of being able to climb the stairs in his house. He and his wife had built their home 35 years earlier when they were younger and healthier. With three stories and two sets of stairs, the house had become increasingly difficult to manage and navigate. Their children suggested that they move somewhere without stairs, but he was reluctant to leave his beloved home. When we evaluated him, he was quite slender, yet his InBody testing demonstrated seriously diminished muscle mass, with fat infiltrating what muscle he had. Here was a clear case of sarcopenia, the wasting away of muscle tissue resulting in progressive weakness and diminished capacity.

Our solution was fourfold. First, we restored his anabolic hormone levels to that of a younger man. Second, we treated him with dasatinib and quercetin for three days each week for three weeks to reduce the number and effect of the senescent cells that were preventing his good cells from growing and reproducing. Third, we put him on an exercise program with a coach at the gym near his home. Fourth, we created a protein-rich diet for him. The major exercise he did at the gym? I bet you guessed it. He worked out a lot on the stair climber.

As expected, he added muscle and strength to his body. The stairs in his home and elsewhere are no longer a challenge. He is a happy and enthusiastic patient, as is his wife, who'd been afraid he was headed for a nursing home and was worried about how she'd cope without him.

Strength Training and Your Joints

When I got my first treadmill and finally improved enough to be able to run rather than walk, as you read in the previous chapter, there were times when my knees protested that they were being abused. I bought neoprene knee sleeves, which added an external bit of stability to minimize wobbles in this inherently unstable joint; slowed down until the pain went away; and then sped up again. Eventually the knee sleeves were no longer needed because my thigh muscles grew strong enough to stabilize my knees and lessen the pain.

It depends on how hard you train, but microtrauma to your muscles when they are being worked triggers healing, not major trauma. You're not trying to rip the joint apart. You are exercising the joint enough to put a little stress on it. This means you should do as much as you comfortably can without pain and without becoming exhausted.

The goal is to develop stronger muscles and ligaments *around* your joints for better support and stabilization. The ligaments and tendons of sedentary people become very weak. Once they start exercising, muscle will grow much faster than ligament and tendon tissue, which grow only about one-third as fast as muscle does. What happens when people increase exercising too quickly is that their muscles become strong, but the ligaments and tendons aren't ready to take the load, so they might rupture or be seriously damaged. They need time to build up.

This is especially true with knees. Like shoulders and elbows, knees are inherently unstable joints. They don't have a ball and a socket like your hips. All that holds the two knee bones together are the muscles that start in your thighs and attach just below the joint on the fibula. These muscles need to be strong enough to pull those ligaments tight to hold the knee joint stable, so it doesn't wobble back and forth, causing pain as you're trying to use it. Every time you step up on a curb or go up the stairs, you're putting *three times your body weight* in force on that cartilage surface, and in order to pull those thigh muscles tight enough, you have to compress that cartilage. People who are overweight often have knee problems because they don't have enough muscle strength to stabilize their knees. Losing just 5 pounds takes 15 pounds of pressure off the cartilage; losing 20 pounds takes 60 pounds of pressure off that cartilage, and so on.

About Arthritis

Are you developing or do you have arthritis? If so, join the 58.5 million Americans (nearly a quarter of all adults) who also have it. Arthritis symptoms include sporadic or chronic pain, swelling, stiffness, and a diminished range of motion in joints. So many people have arthritis that it is now the leading cause of disability in this country.

Arthritis isn't just a condition that targets seniors; it can develop at any age, most commonly starting after the age of 40. The most common form is osteoarthritis, which is found in knees, hips, the spine, and hands. (Rheumatoid arthritis is an autoimmune disease.)

Arthritis is one of those conditions that is a perfect example of doctors needing to rethink what they learned in medical school. Read this statement from the Arthritis Foundation—the italics are mine, for emphasis—and you'll understand what I mean. They explain that osteoarthritis is "a disease of the whole joint, not just cartilage. Bones in affected joints become weaker, the connective tissue that holds the joint together deteriorates, and inflammation damages the joint lining. *Contrary to decades of belief*, inflammation plays a key role in osteoarthritis, just as it does in most other types of arthritis."

There's that pesky word again: *inflammation*. When I was a young medical student, we thought that the reason overweight people developed joint problems was their weight. We were partially right. It is fat that triggers the systemic inflammatory products that lead to joint destruction. Since fat accounts for most of the extra weight, it is fat that causes the problem, but not by the mechanism that we once believed.

Stretching and Your Joints

Stretching is something that is easy to do and can feel so good. A lot of people don't stretch because they've got this notion that it's annoying, painful, or unnecessary. Instead, I'd like you to think of stretching as your version of the languid movements that cats and dogs make when they wake up from a nap. They clearly like to stretch!

Doing a few stretches only takes a couple of minutes. You can do them at home at any time and at no cost. If you want to use stretch bands, they cost a few dollars. With stretching, you will quickly get results and see improvements. The more you stretch, the easier it becomes as your range of motion increases.

My Morning Stretch Routine

I have a simple and quick stretching routine that I do every morning.

- After I shave, I do a few squats. I then twist my shoulders as comfortably as I can to the left, then to the right three or four times.
- I bend forward to place my hands flat on the floor with my knees locked—an extension of touching your toes. I bend further down three or four times to stretch my back and hamstrings.
- Then I reach toward the ceiling and rotate my shoulders through a full range of motion.
- I drop to the floor and knock out my push-ups.
- I make our bed. This has nothing to do with my stretching, even though you do have to reach to make a bed properly. It's just the one household chore that my wife does not enjoy, so I do it. Use this as a reminder that doing chores is exercise, so don't forget to add those steps and movements when tracking your activity.

Fit your stretching routine into your day just as you make time for your cardio and strength training. If you work at a desk, set a timer and get up at least once or twice an hour and do a minute or two of stretches; ditto on an airplane. Or when waiting for an elevator, use the wall to stretch against. Sometimes when taking my walk around the block, I will stop and squat and stretch. I don't care if someone sees me and rolls their eyes. I know what feels wonderful and they don't!

When I'm back in the office, I do these same stretch squats multiple times during the day. I can't squat down very deeply because of the hand grenade that damaged my left knee when I fought in Vietnam. Instead, I bend down and put my hands flat on the floor to stretch. This puts a good but not painful strain on my lower back, hips, and knees. I do this about six times. I do a great hamstring stretch by simply bending over and placing my palms flat on the floor. If you wish, you can cross your legs before you bend down to take some of the strain off your back.

About Yoga and Pilates

When I was growing up, yoga was practiced by few people in this country. Now, it's incredibly popular, with yoga studios everywhere. As yoga combines physical movement in the form of poses (known as asanas) with controlled breathing and a meditative aspect, it can be deeply satisfying for both body and soul, improving overall health as well as strengthening and adding enormous flexibility to your joints.

There are many different types of yoga. For instance, hot yoga is done in a heated room that makes you start sweating immediately. I prefer the most mellow and light kind of yoga that is primarily about gentle stretching. Hatha yoga is often recommended for seniors as it is done slowly. You can even do yoga poses in a chair rather than on the floor if your mobility is limited. Some classes add aerobic movements and challenging poses to the mix to get your heart rate up. I don't recommend this style of yoga unless you are already a seasoned exerciser, because it can easily cause injuries.

Pilates is a form of exercise invented by a German trainer named Joseph Pilates. (He originally called it Contrology.) It is especially valuable for strengthening all the core muscles effectively, which helps improve posture, support your spine, and tighten up core muscles. Pilates complements any other exercise routines you do, even yoga. It can be done at home but is most effective when done under supervision in a dedicated studio by a trained instructor. There are exercises done on mats and specific Pilates equipment, notably the Reformer, that target particular muscles.

With either yoga or Pilates, never push yourself into a pose that gives you even a twinge of pain. You should feel calm yet energized after a yoga or Pilates session—not sore and fed up!

To Move Faster and with More Stability, Do Balance Training

No matter your age and how fit you are, everyone needs balance training. When you have enough strength in your extremities, this will help keep you from getting injured. You will also have confidence in your ability to move without worrying about falling.

Balance is a matter of *proprioception*, which is the awareness of your body in physical space. It gives you coordination, so you automatically use it when, for example, you are walking down a crowded street and your body knows how to avoid bumping into people. Those proprioceptors are sensory fibers that let you know exactly what your feet and legs are doing and where they are at any given moment without having to look and see them. As we age, we lose both the number and sensitivity of these nerve endings, and this in turn impacts our balance and sensory awareness. In the worst case scenario, the brain, which is already shrinking with age, starts losing track of what our feet, ankles, knees, and hips are doing at any given moment, so we trip and stumble on uneven surfaces or even over minor impediments on the ground if we're not consciously paying attention or get distracted while walking. This is one of the reasons seniors lose their balance and frequently fall down.

The good news is that you can counteract diminished proprioception to some degree with balance training. Also, check out your local senior center or Y, as many of them have balance classes that can be of tremendous help.

The Danger of Falls as You Get Older

Accidents happen. As I detailed in the previous chapter, one day I was walking along, trying to put the code in my phone, when I tripped over the curb and smashed up my shoulder. Who was to blame? Me. We know that looking at your phone while you're walking anywhere is stupid! Stupidity has consequences, and we're all stupid from time to time. Sometimes we get away with it, and sometimes it bites us right in the rump—or in my case, in the shoulder.

When accidents happen, it's either due to our not paying attention or it's due to bad luck. It's Rule #15: You can do everything right and things can still go to hell. When I lived in Utah, I fell lots of times when going to see patients thanks to the slick black ice that I could not see. I was fortunate that I never broke any bones!

A similar fall now could be catastrophic for someone my age, even at my level of fitness. According to the National Institutes of Health, "Hip fracture among older patients is a devastating injury in most cases. It profoundly affects the physical, mental, functional, and social balance that patients used to have and, beyond the orthopedic injury, it reflects the aging process and its dire consequences. Some reports show that up to 50 percent of patients with hip fracture die within six months and many of those who survive do not recover their baseline independence and function. In recent decades the increase in life expectancy after 60 years of age has led to an exponential growth in hip fractures."

In fact, 25 percent of those with the kind of hip fracture I wrote about at the beginning of this chapter never live independently again unless they get a hip replacement; they're disabled and need a wheelchair because the bone itself never completely heals after its blood supply is affected.

Broken hips are notorious for sending people to nursing homes—and you don't want that to be you!

For some with a hip fracture, a total hip replacement might be an option, but it is a difficult and major operation that requires months of physical therapy afterward. As you know, all major surgery carries risks. Even if you fall and don't break a bone, it can take a long time to heal and recuperate as you age. Damage to tendons and ligaments can take even longer—often many months—to heal.

That's why those "I've fallen and I can't get up" devices are worth exploring if you have balance issues. They remove some of the fear and anxiety, especially if you live alone, that you won't be able to call for help. I gave one to my mother, and one day I got an alert and instantly panicked. "Did you fall? What hurts?" I asked. "Oh no," she said, "I'm going to the gym, and I just got lost. I need directions." (My mom was 88 at this point.) "Mom," I replied, "you just finished a trip around the world on your own. You set foot on every continent on earth, and you got turned around going to the gym?" This did concern me because getting lost is often a sign of early dementia, and given her age, I had to consider the possibility. But we just laughed this time. She was fine.

The great thing about balance training is that progress is quick—and that's wonderfully gratifying. Most people will do balance exercises only for seconds, not minutes. If you can find five minutes in your day to do these exercises, you will see an amazing difference in a week.

How to Do Balance Training

Preventing falls is a matter of balance, coordination, and strength.

When I was a paratrooper, I knew how to fall. We trained hard for it. But that was a planned fall when I knew that the ground was coming up and learned how to prepare to get into position. An accidental fall, on the other hand, happens so quickly that adrenaline kicks in and you won't realize what's happening until it's over. Even if you're trained as I was, you won't be able to run through a checklist before you hit the ground!

Balance exercises help improve the ability to stay in control of body movement and to correct yourself when you lose your balance. How much balance training you need depends on your strength and how unstable you are. You need to balance enough so that you can stand like a stork without wavering or falling:

- Stand on one leg, then put one foot up by the inside or the outside of your knee.
- Keep standing on that one leg for as long as you can.
- Repeat with the other leg and stay there for a while.

Note: If you're just starting out, stand next to or hold onto a chair for stability. The goal is to build up muscle strength to be able to do a stork without support.

Balance Training Exercises

- Stork: Do this for as long as you can as described on page 151.
- Standing Balance Alphabet: Stand on one leg on a firm surface. Using your non-support foot, "write" the alphabet in cursive. Repeat with the other leg. Eventually you will get up to Z!
- Standing Balance with a Ball: Stand on one leg, have someone throw you a ball, and catch it. Repeat with the other leg.
- Sitting Balance: Sit up straight in a firm chair with armrests. Extend one leg out, then hold onto the armrests and close your eyes. Repeat on the other side.

Note: The following walks become progressively more difficult.

- Heel-to-Toe Walk #1: Walk heel to toe, with your arms spread out at shoulder height for stability.
- Heel-to-Toe Walk #2: Do #1 while adding on a cognitive task, such as counting backwards in multiples of four.

- Heel-to-Toe Walk #3: Do #1 with the lights dimmed or while wearing sunglasses.
- Heel-to-Toe Walk #4: Do #1 with your arms at your sides or folded across your chest.
- Heel-to-Toe Walk #5: Do #1 with your eyes closed.
- Heel-to-Toe Walk #6: Do #1 while turning your head from side to side, with your arms spread out at shoulder height for stability. As you progress, keep your arms at your sides or folded across your chest.

Here are some more balance training tips:

- Once you've mastered the stork and can stand on one foot for two minutes, do it with your eyes closed. Keep that chair handy when you start, as I can guarantee that you will be wavering, and your foot will quickly come down! Doing any balance exercise with your eyes closed is an excellent way to improve, since you won't be relying on visual proprioception and will be using only your muscle strength and the cues built into your ears and muscles instead.
- Be sure to keep your core muscles tight during these exercises by keeping your buttocks squeezed and your belly button pulled to your spine. Doing so will help you prevent injury and maintain your balance.
- Never hold your breath.
- As with stretching, you can take breaks to do balance training throughout the day. Do them when you're on the phone or waiting for the elevator or the bus. Just be sure you have something sturdy nearby to hold on to.
- If you can do longer balance sessions several times per week, for up to 20 minutes per session, you will make amazing progress. Ideally, you

should do longer sessions after your body is warmed up with cardiovascular exercise, followed by strength training and stretching.

- Do balance exercises when you're alert and not tired. For optimal results, your nervous system needs to be well rested.

Note: For more about balance training and your brain, go to page 218 in Chapter 9.

Recommended Supplements for Moving Faster

Refer to Chapter 5 for more details. Discuss the proper doses for your needs as well as any potential contraindications with your doctor before taking any new supplements.

Astaxanthin This is the reddish-orange pigment in salmon. It is a powerful muscle booster that allows salmon to swim upstream against the current and jump up waterfalls to get to their spawning grounds. A study at the University of Washington demonstrated that 10 mg a day of astaxanthin increased strength and endurance in older men and women.

Creatine See page 160 for more information.

Vitamin D3 and Vitamin K2 The combined actions of vitamins D3 and K2 lead to enhanced immune response, denser bones, and improved emotional stability. Because these two vitamins synergize, they are often sold as one supplement for more effective absorption. The advantage of the K2 over regular vitamin K is that it does not counteract the anticlotting drugs that many people take.

Chapter 8
Leaner

When I was Fat Jerry and working 14 hours a day as a country doctor, I rarely ate a meal at home. I chowed down at the nearby Mexican restaurant for lunch and snacked all day long. When I took a break, I'd go to Safeway, buy the fresh-from-the-oven cheese-walnut-raisin bread, and eat the entire loaf in one sitting. After work, I staggered home, totally exhausted, had a snack, fell into bed, and started all over again the next day. At 49, I was divorced and virtually sexless. I felt old, tired, and fat and was so depressed I could barely function.

Something had to change. I started doing research to figure out what was happening to me. I quickly discovered #1 on my list: I needed to become lean, and #2, as you read in the previous two chapters, I needed to become fit. Lean and fit. That became my new mantra.

But how was I going to do that when I ate and ate all day long? It wasn't just me. I looked around and realized that America has the fattest population of the world's developed nations. I read about how our life spans are falling when they should be rising. About how many diseases are connected to being overweight, thanks to destructive pro-inflammatory fat production. Dementia has almost doubled; diabetes tripled; heart disease has gone up 270 percent; osteoporosis and degenerative joint disease increased; and 22 percent of all cancers in America are caused by being overweight. It's that visceral fat kicking out inflammatory cytokines throughout your whole body and killing your brain, your heart, your joints, your pancreas, your muscles.

What were we doing wrong? What could I do about it? Let me tell you. . . .

The Chubbies Inherited the Earth

Why We Get Fat

Back in our cave-dwelling days, when it came to animals, human beings were puny in tooth and claw—hunter/gatherers who were a lot better at gathering than hunting. Our ancestors knew they'd lose a fight with a 40-pound bobcat that could easily kill them. So our ancestors were scavenger/gatherers, eating mainly fruits, berries, nuts, seeds, roots, vegetables, and leaves because they don't run very fast! They were intermittent eaters—scarfing down whatever was available. If it wasn't available, they didn't eat. They starved and died instead. Our ancestors did their best to stuff themselves in the summer and fall when grains, grasses, and fruits were available. They knew that winter was coming and food was going to be in short supply. If they went into winter skinny, chances were good that they wouldn't survive to reproduce the next year. That left Mother Nature seriously displeased.

That's why the chubbies inherited the earth. Only those who put on every pound of fat they possibly could would live through the winter and have babies. Those who were genetically coded to become the fattest the fastest in a short summer/fall period were the ones who survived unforgiving winters.

We now carry that same genome with us. We've been coded to crave fattier, richer, sweeter, and more energy-packed food. We crave it and we are designed to eat as much of it as is available. But our ancestors' survival traits are what's killing us today, because high-fat, high-sugar foods are available 24/7 everywhere in America. Factor in how food manufacturers know the exact ratio to get us addicted to their combos of salt, sugar, and fat and it's no wonder the chubbies are everywhere you look.

As I said in the introduction, it is *not* a moral failing to be fat. It doesn't make you a bad person; it makes you bad at planning your meals.

Because all you're doing is giving in to what your genetics are telling you to do. When doctors tell people to lose weight, they're asking them to do an inherently unnatural act.

We can't change what we are since it's built into our genome—but we can restructure our livestyles to maximize calorie burn and muscle production while minimizing fat production and cravings for calorie-dense junk food. We need to look for ways to alter our lives and make them less destructive. It's not about going on a fad diet. It's about having a better mindset about food for the rest of our days so we can become successful at losing and maintaining an ideal weight.

How Much Should I Weigh?

Although I addressed this earlier, it bears repeating: When patients ask me, "How much should I weigh?" my answer is always the same: "I don't know!" I can't tell patients what they should weigh because human beings have an incredible amount of variation in body type. There are people designed to be lean, tall willows, while others are fireplugs. There are people meant to be broad and thick, others fine-boned and petite.

But I do suggest that they take Dr. Mixon's Jiggle Test to get a better idea.

Dr. Mixon's Jiggle Test

Take off all your clothes, stand in front of a mirror, and jump up and down. Anything that jiggles other than breasts on women and genitals on men should not be there. You should be lean and firm.

Body mass index, or BMI, is a standard measurement for weight. But it's a bit of a false marker. According to the CDC, a BMI less than 18.5 means you're underweight; 18.5 to 24.9 is a healthy weight range; 25.0 to 29.9 is overweight; and 30.0 or higher is obese. But your BMI only measures surface area to height; it can't differentiate between fat and muscle.

(Muscle weighs more than fat.) My BMI tells me I should lose 30 pounds, which would leave me emaciated!

A much better measurement is with a device we use in our clinics called InBody. It measures the percentage of muscle and fat in your legs, arms, and torso. It's especially important to know your torso measurements because visceral fat is so destructive. As you age, strands of fat infiltrate your muscles, making them weaker. (This is one of the reasons seniors often have such weak muscles.)

Do Weight Loss Medications Work?

If any one weight loss medication worked well, obesity levels would go way, way down. Contrary to all those ads for "Burn fat overnight!" pills and gummies, there are limited pharmaceutical options when it comes to weight loss. All of them have side effects, which can be gross at best and horrendous at worst.

If you're wondering why so many previously overweight celebrities are suddenly thin and trim, it's not because they upped their workouts. Rather it's due to a new class of prescription weight loss meds, originally developed to treat diabetes, that lower blood glucose levels and hunger signals. These medications include Mounjaro, Wegovy, and Ozempic. They take off weight quickly because you lose your appetite, but side effects include nausea, diarrhea, other gastrointestinal problems, and hair loss. And when you stop taking the medication, you quickly regain the weight because you're ravenous and overeat. (These medications are also very expensive, costing more than $1,000 per month and are rarely covered by insurance.) If you are pre-diabetic, diabetic, and/or obese and want to try one of them, discuss this with your doctor, as the positives in reducing inflammation and insulin resistance for those who truly need help may outweigh the negatives. Recognize, however, that when you've lost the weight, you're probably going to still need this medication at least one week out of every month to keep it off, which will reduce the cost, but may still give you the unwelcome side effects.

There are several other weight loss drugs that prevent you from absorbing fat. I don't recommend them as they tend to give people uncontrollable diarrhea. You can also become deficient in the fat-soluble vitamins your brain and body need.

In our clinics, we sometimes use a prescription drug called phentermine hydrochloride to help jump-start treatment for obese patients. This drug was popular back in the 1980s when it was sold with another drug, fenfluramine, in a combo called fen-phen, but fenfluramine caused heart valve and other heart problems. Phentermine, on the other hand, is a mild amphetamine and, if used carefully, is an effective appetite suppressant that also keeps you wide awake and alert. The usual dose is to take it every day for seven to ten days, and after that never more than three days a week to prevent addiction. I tell patients that if they don't need it three times a week, don't take it. Save it for days when you wake up and you know it's going to be a big eating day—a business dinner that night or a holiday event. This drug isn't meant to be used long-term. It's a jump-start. The idea is to take it for a month or two to help you retrain your eating patterns. Use it in conjunction with adding healthier, fiber-rich foods to your meals and controlling portion sizes.

Slow and Steady Weight Loss Is the Only Way to Lose Pounds and Keep Them Off

Yo-yos are toys for playing with, not for dieting!

On a typical diet, people starve themselves for a few weeks or suffer through highly restrictive meals. They lose a few pounds, but in the meantime their metabolism slows down in response to fewer calories. When the dieting stops, their metabolism doesn't speed up again, the pounds quickly come back, and it becomes harder to lose them again. Cutting calories for just four days reduces blood levels of leptin (the "I'm full" hormone) by 40 percent, which makes you hungrier and even less likely to stick to a diet.

Many of us are stress eaters. We find food comforting, and sometimes turn to it like a reliable friend to make us feel better when times are tough. We use food like alcoholics use booze. The difference is that while abstinence is a practical means of avoiding overindulgence in alcohol, we all need to eat to survive.

The reality is that there is no one best diet that works for everyone. There are plenty of severe and destructive diets, even some that make your body start eating its own muscle. We each have personalities, strengths, weaknesses, and idiosyncrasies that keep any one diet from fitting all of our needs. The one consistent factor in successful weight loss programs is accountability and making the lifestyle changes I keep mentioning.

The bottom line: You can't lose weight and keep it off if you don't exercise and improve your muscle strength at the same time. When you add lots of dietary fiber and techniques to stop overeating along with improved hormone levels that make muscle, your body is less likely to turn extra calories into fat. Remember, thanks to Mother Nature, fat is our default tissue, instead of the muscle that's a high-energy-consuming tissue.

Mother Nature sure loves her chubbies!

One Pound a Week Is the Way to Go

When I talk to people about weight loss, I tell them that they're not going to lose 30 pounds in the next month. Four pounds a month, one pound a week, is the way to go. Start simple.

Here's the formula: There are about 3,500 calories in one pound of fat. If you reduce your calorie intake by 500 calories a day, that equals one pound a week. A slice of bread has 100 calories, so if you take the bread off one sandwich a day, that's 200 calories. And if you up your exercise by 300 calories, bingo! You've got your 500 calories a day. Or, you can cut your eating by 300 calories and increase your exercise by 200 calories to reach 500 calories a day. That's one pound a week, or 50 pounds a year. That's an achievable and sustainable goal.

Use Your Workout Time Effectively to Reduce Your Appetite

Men have enormous advantages over women when it comes to losing weight. We have naturally higher muscle mass that burns calories 24/7, even when at rest or asleep.

Eighty percent of men lose their appetites with vigorous exercise. (Not a leisurely stroll with the dog, but a workout that makes you sweat.) Why is that? No one knows. The other 20 percent stimulate their appetites with exercise. On the other hand, only 50 percent of women lose their appetites when they exercise. The other half are ravenous after a workout. Which one are you?

- If your appetite is suppressed by exercise, exercise when you're hungry. You'll not only burn calories, but you will be less inclined to eat more when you're done with your workout.
- If exercise increases your appetite, you *might* want to reward yourself after jogging with a 500-calorie smoothie. Instead, eat before you work out.
- The more you work out to take advantage of this pattern, the easier you'll be able to control your eating over time.

Let's Talk About Fad Diets

One of the most important things I've learned as a physician is that just because it was true 20 years ago doesn't mean that's the case now. Eggs are bad! Oh wait, no, they're good for you. Artificial sweeteners will curb those sugar cravings! Um, nope. Your body processes them as if they were real sugar. Fat-free is the way to go! Sure, if you want to put on weight eating foods that replace fat with sugar.

When the high-fat, super-low-carb Atkins diet was the rage in the 1990s, people jumped on the trend wagon, lost weight, and often became sick. They went off the diet, gained the weight back, plus more, and then spent a lifetime thinking of healthy carbs as the enemy.

The most successful diet book I ever read was written by cardiologist Dean Ornish. He originally wrote it to help people open up their coronary arteries and reverse heart disease solely with dietary change. Nobody bought it until his publisher had the brilliant idea of retitling it *Eat More, Weigh Less*, because one of the side effects of his system was weight loss. The book was a bestseller for years. The diet is now outdated because it is very low in fat—so low in fat that it would pull the plaque out of your arteries. I tried the diet for six months and became the leanest I'd ever been in my life. I went off it when a new girlfriend who loved to cook entered my life for a bit, and I never mustered the near religious fervor needed to go back on it. The diet does make you lose weight and lowers arterial plaque, but you need to be a bit of a fanatic to stick with such restrictive eating. Most of us can only work up that degree of enthusiasm for brief periods.

Can the Keto Diet Help Me Lose Weight?

Look online or on bookshelves and you'll be confronted with *The Paleo Diet*, *The South Beach Diet*, *Becoming Vegan*, *The Zone Diet*, *The Dash Diet*, and more. But let's talk about what the keto diet is.

I remember my first patient from my country doctor days who was diabetic and put himself on a ketogenic diet. In those days, I recommended the American Diabetes Association's diets for my diabetic patients. After all, they were the experts, so why argue? Anyway, this fellow, who'd been my patient for years, came in and said, "Doc, I was having trouble with my sugars, so I went on this here keto diet and my sugars are fabulous." I ran his blood work, and he was right. It was a revelation to me that perhaps the American Diabetes Association didn't know what it was talking about. Maybe this off-the-wall diet that according to my training should have given my patient heart attacks, strokes, and clogged arteries had potential. I had to be humble enough to realize my patient might know something I didn't.

I started reading about ketogenic diets, long before they were popular. Ketosis is a condition we develop when our body burns fat instead of glucose; ketone bodies are produced whether the fat comes from your food or from your belly.

Like the Atkins diet, the keto diet is a high-fat, low-carb plan that throws your body into ketosis. For the short term (three to four months), I have no objections if you do follow this diet for weight loss. Bear in mind, however, that it can make you feel awful (aka the keto flu), with low energy. This can lead to curtailed workouts, which isn't a good idea. To track whether or not you're producing ketones and burning fat, you can buy ketone testing strips at the drugstore—dip one in a urine specimen for an instant result. If you're not producing ketones, you're not burning fat, and you need to alter what you're eating or how much you're eating if you want to lose weight.

In the long term, however, the keto diet adds huge amounts of fat and cholesterol to your body. You already know that cholesterol is not the demon it's made out to be. It's the mother hormone, necessary for cell metabolism that keeps your brain, muscles, and heart working. But the more cholesterol in your system, the higher the risk of forming plaque in your arteries that can contribute to heart attacks and strokes. Whenever you're eating lots and lots of fat—red meat and full-fat dairy products—you're eating lots of cholesterol. If that happens, you want to make sure you're also eating fruits and vegetables with lots of antioxidants so you don't develop free radicals. Keep your energy expenditure high enough so you don't drive your insulin too high, which will send your sugar load skyrocketing. In addition, the keto diet is absurdly low in the fiber you need because it's almost all animal protein, and fiber is largely comes from vegetables and grains.

If you wash down a keto meal with a Coke or have dessert, you have the worst of both worlds: Those enormous amounts of fat and cholesterol zooming right along your digestive system, topped with a gigantic sugar load. When that happens, Mother Nature is laughing all the way to the tempting new French bakery that just opened up, and you're paying the price.

An Unusual Case

Although most people who come to our clinics are overweight, we are sometimes approached by our patients asking that we consult with their children or grandchildren for an endocrine-related problem. I have a surgeon friend who jokingly claims that my clinic has become a mecca for "cosmetic endocrinology." I am not all that happy with such a description since we do not normally address endocrine diseases. Our focus is on correcting what "normally" happens to impair our health and happiness.

Still, I was surprised when a patient asked us to consult about her 16-year-old anorexic granddaughter, who weighed a shockingly low 70 pounds. The fear was that she might die at any moment. We discussed the request in our weekly rounds and one of our doctors, a warm and loving grandmother herself, begged permission to try to help the girl. She arranged for her to be seen weekly by an adolescent psychiatrist as well as her family doctor, with us as consultants. Since the patient's self-imposed starvation had shut down her hormone production, she was producing almost no estrogen, progesterone, testosterone, thyroid, DHEA, or pregnenolone. We boosted all of her deficient hormones to mid-adolescent levels, which made her hungry as all get-out, and provided additional tools to improve her health. The psychiatrist, her family doctor, and our physician effectively granny-loved her back toward health. This isn't what we usually do, but it sure made me feel good.

How to Eat for Longevity

Dr. Mixon's Golden Rules of Eating

1. Recognize the signs of true hunger. Eat only when you're really hungry, not out of habit—and toss those nighttime snacks.
2. Eat your biggest meals early in the day.
3. Downsize those super-sized portions by at least half.
4. Fiber is your friend.
5. Fat is a part-time friend.
6. Sugar is not your friend.

7. The brighter the colors, the better the nutrients.

8. Put vegetables and salads at the center of your plate, with smaller servings of protein, especially red meat.

1. Recognize the signs of true hunger. eat only when you're really hungry, not out of habit—and toss those nighttime snacks.

Eat less food, less frequently. I know you can do it.

The feeling of an empty stomach isn't an emergency! Learn that when your tummy growls, it doesn't mean you need to eat immediately. Most people (diabetics excluded) can go a long time without eating every single day. You won't starve. You are going to be just fine.

If you're overweight, teach yourself to eat less than your body craves. If you are one of those lucky people for whom exercise dampens your appetite, you should work out at those times when you'll otherwise be snacking. You'll pass that time exercising and you'll lose your appetite, which helps a lot.

Eating at night before going to bed is guaranteed to stymie your weight loss and is the biggest weight control mistake you can make. Going to bed hungry causes your metabolism to drop to its lowest point of the day while you're asleep. Any food still in your gut will take hours to digest, and the energy it generates can't be burned off. Instead, it's converted to fat and stored for later use. If, on the other hand, you go to bed with an empty gut, you may hear that rumbling, but you won't die before the sun rises. By not eating at night, your body will burn that glycogen in your liver, use it for fuel, and burn fat instead.

In other words, every single night of your life you are going to either make fat (because you have food in your gut) or burn fat (because your gut is empty). That's part of why intermittent fasting works, as I'll explain on page 188.

Another way to lessen your cravings for nighttime snacking is to take an evening walk or do some modest exercise after you eat. Such a walk is called a "constitutional" for a reason—because it's good for your constitution! You'll not only burn off more of those calories, but you'll improve your digestion by increasing the peristalsis (movement) of your gastrointestinal tract. This will push waste through faster and make you less likely to be constipated.

If I wake up at two in the morning and my tummy is screaming, *Why don't you get up and eat?* I tell it to shut up and I go back to sleep!

2. Eat your biggest meals early in the day.

The typical Western meal pattern is topsy-turvy. Instead, as the saying goes, you should eat like a king at breakfast, a prince at lunch, and a pauper at dinner.

Breakfast I've never understood the appeal of eating sweet cereals, bagels, toast, or pancakes—aside from convenience—first thing in the morning. They're simple carbohydrates that are quickly digested and leave you hungry a scant hour or two later. It's much better to eat a substantial meal that includes protein and complex carbohydrates for that early morning energy boost. A protein load will push you through until lunch, jump-starting your metabolism and preventing energy sags later in the day. If you are a man, your testosterone levels peak at about 8 a.m. and reach their lowest points during the early evening. By timing your biggest meal in the morning, you capitalize on that surge of metabolic power.

Lunch This should be your midsized meal. Again, it needs a good mix of complex carbohydrates and protein to carry you through the afternoon and into the early evening.

Dinner The evening meal should be your smallest meal of the day, and it should be consumed early enough in the evening—at least two or three hours before bedtime—to give you an almost empty stomach at bedtime. See #1 above!

Snacks Small and hardly ever is the way to go. I do enjoy the occasional ice cream cone on a hot day while on vacation. No, I do not eat a big bowl of ice cream each evening in front of the TV. I have a friend who jokes that snacks have their own four food groups: crunchy, chewy, bacon, and chocolate.

- If you like crunchy: Try air-popped popcorn instead of chips, or a small handful of nuts or seeds. If you crack your own sunflower seeds, you won't be done snacking quickly because they're such a pain to open!
- If you like chewy: Try a small amount (no more than ¼ to ½ cup) of dried fruit, frozen berries, or grapes instead of candy. While dried fruit has a lot of fructose and calories, it also contains lots of fiber.
- If you like bacon: Try beef jerky instead. It's low in calories and takes a long time to chew.
- If you like chocolate: Dark chocolate contains antioxidants and many different minerals. Just a small square.

Intermittent Fasting

I've found one of the best ways to manage my appetite and deal with Rule #1 and #2 is intermittent fasting. This eating methods means you eat only within specified periods, and drink only non-caloric liquids outside of that period. I rarely eat after lunch, although I may put that meal off until 2 or 3 p.m. (Is that *lunner* or *dunch*?) I eat again early the next morning. The timing works out to be 16:8 (16 hours of not eating with an 8-hour window for meals). Many people prefer 14:10 (14 hours of not eating, 10 hours for meals) because it's easier to manage.

Intermittent fasting not only curbs your appetite and helps you realize when you're truly hungry, it also allows your body to alter your immune response to an anti-inflammatory mode. It increases autophagy, the process by which you replace worn and damaged cells with fresh, healthy ones. Decades of animal studies have shown that intermittent fasting, which more closely mimics the intermittent eating habits of our remote ancestors, has beneficial effect on our whole metabolism. (A side effect in animals that are trained to fast intermittently is that their life span is extended. Even more important is that their health span, the length of time during which they are strong, healthy, robust, and able to enjoy a high quality of life, is also extended.)

Changing the way you eat is not a quick process. Intermittent fasting can be difficult for those who like to eat small meals and snacks throughout the day. It's not recommended for diabetics, who must eat at regular intervals to maintain their glucose levels. (If you are diabetic or pre-diabetic, always consult your doctor before changing the timing of your meals.) Cut yourself some slack and take your time getting used to it. Some people adjust quickly, while others take weeks or even months to gradually increase the time between the last meal of the day and the first one the next morning. Of course, there will be evenings when you have family events, business meetings, or you're just hanging out with friends and you want to eat and join in. Go for it! Just delay your breakfast the next morning or start all over the day after that. It doesn't much matter when you fast as long as you do the fasting. Adapt it to your needs.

And stop thinking that a grumbling stomach means you must feed it right this minute.

How I Eat Every Day

Because I don't eat dinner, I wake up ravenous and stumble into the kitchen by 5:45 a.m. for breakfast. Since I follow the eat like a king at breakfast/prince at lunch/pauper at dinner philosophy, my breakfast is three or four eggs, toast, butter, some bacon or ham, a few veggies, whipped cream (I really do need the fat!), peanut butter, jam, and black coffee. And yes, I eat every morsel! After I'm finished, I go out for my morning trail jog for a few miles. By the time I get back home, Banding has a 12-ounce cappuccino with some chocolate and sprinkles on top ready for me.

I eat lunch with my executive team. It's usually a combination of salad greens with some chicken or pork. I often take home a box of leftovers to use in an omelet the next morning.

For snacks in the morning, I might have a handful of nuts or a single square of dark chocolate. I don't snack after lunch; my body knows I'm done for the day!

3. Downsize those super-sized portions by at least half.

One night, not long after my Chinese-born wife Banding first came to America, she had a craving for a milkshake. I took her to Dairy Queen for a Blizzard, and she insisted that we buy a medium-sized one. When we got home, she took out two spoons. After we each had about three bites, she said, "Okay, that's enough. Put the lid on and put it in the freezer." I was bewildered. In my world, when you bought a Blizzard, you ate the entire Blizzard. In her world, you bought a Blizzard and ate it over a week, with two bites a night. "But we only got one Blizzard for two people, and we barely touched it!" I protested.

"Well, she said with a smile, "You don't need that much. *You just need to know what it tastes like.*"

That was my introduction to my wife's philosophy about eating. I quickly came to appreciate the wisdom of her approach to eating as opposed to my own early gluttony. She taught me that you really do not need to eat the whole damn thing, which is why it's been decades since I've eaten an entire Blizzard in one sitting.

When you do lose your appetite, you realize how little food you do need to eat to survive. Again, this is not a moral failure as practically everything in America has been super-sized since I was growing up. Back then, a bottle of Coke was six ounces. It cost a nickel, and you had to drink it right away because the glass bottle had to be recycled back into the wooden box they put outside the store. Today, a can of Coke is 12 ounces and costs a dollar or more.

It's hard to gauge what an appropriate portion size should be now. If you look at the label on a box of pasta, one serving of pasta is two ounces (200 calories). Nobody eats just two ounces of pasta. If you order pasta in a restaurant, you're likely to be served at least eight ounces. Look at the calorie count at the Olive Garden for a serving of their chicken Alfredo pasta. It has 1,570 calories. A little less than what an average-sized woman needs to eat for the *entire day.*

You want to eat as much as your body needs, no more. (If you want the chicken Alfredo, ask for a takeout box when you place your order. Immediately put half of it in the box for another meal.) One bit of advice I sometimes give patients is that if they want to see what a proper portion size is, sign up for NutriSystem's introductory packet. They'll send you a box containing everything you're supposed to eat for a month. You will be shocked when you see what serving sizes should look like. Also, think of airline food portions. They look much smaller than we're used to because we've been taught to expect super-sized portions.

When my family goes out to eat, Banding and I usually order one salad and one savory entrée, plus an appetizer for Ivory, our fit and active 11-year-old daughter. This is more than enough food for the three of us and we often take some home. The portions are just too large for our needs.

4. Fiber is your friend.

Fiber is the primary prebiotic that gives us great gut health. When mixed with water, fiber fills your stomach and slows the rate your stomach empties, so those hunger rumblings stop.

Fiber is more than just a space saver to decrease your appetite; it also has a metabolic function in your gut. When fiber hits the duodenum, the small intestine below your stomach, it sends signals to your brain to change the way you process carbohydrates by releasing gut hormones called incretins. These are triggered to reduce insulin resistance and the absorption of sugars, slowing the transit and metabolism of carbohydrates. By processing food more slowly, you lower your insulin levels, which is a good thing. This also makes the total calorie count going into your system lower than the total amount of calories you ate.

In addition, soluble fiber is fermented in the gut to a variety of compounds that offer protection in several ways. Some of these bond to both fat and cholesterol, inhibiting their absorption through the bowel wall, so you absorb fewer calories and less fat from your diet. It helps to create a better cholesterol ratio by raising your HDL levels and lowering your LDL and triglyceride levels. It improves your intestinal transit time, softening stools and increasing bulk, thereby reducing the risk of colon cancer.

Your Microbiome Needs That Fiber!

A fascinating study published in the journal *Nature* in June 2023 showed that high-fiber foods are primarily digested in the large intestine, where your microbiome can feed on them and thrive. Low-fiber processed foods are largely digested in the small intestine, which then absorbs nearly all the calories. This can explain why not all calories are equal, and why it's so hard to lose weight even if you're not eating a lot—the fiber quantity/quality of the food is all-important. Junk calories turn into the glucose you don't need, which leads to insulin resistance and fat; fiber-rich foods give you fewer calories, as much of their content is non-digestible and excreted.

High-calorie foods tend to be low in fiber. Our ancestors got their fiber from vegetables, nuts, berries, and unrefined whole grains. Today, many people would rather eat white bread and pasta than beans, legumes, whole grains, and brown rice. They peel the skins off potatoes and fruit, which is where the fiber is concentrated.

If you just can't stand the taste or texture of fiber-rich foods, take a daily fiber supplement. Almost everyone can tolerate two or three Fibercon capsules or the recommended dose of Metamucil. Take either of these supplements before meals so when you start eating, your tummy is already partly full. This especially useful as we get older, because one downside of aging is we lose the feeling that we've had enough to eat. As your satiety sensors decrease, you tend to eat more until you feel stuffed. When you're stuffed it means you've eaten too much!

5. Fat is a part-time friend.

Your brain needs good fats, the omega-3 kind found in fatty fish (salmon, tuna, and sardines), seaweed, green veggies, avocados, and more. Your body needs these good fats for basic metabolic needs and to process fat-soluble vitamins. Your skin needs good fats to produce the oils that provide hydration.

But as you learned in Chapter 3, the more visceral fat you have, the more likely you are to develop serious health problems over time that can make a serious dent in your longevity. That doesn't mean you stop eating fats and eat only fat-free foods that are loaded with sugar. Too much sugar leads to insulin resistance and will shift your metabolism toward fat.

6. Sugar is not your friend.

Mother Nature pulled another whammy by making breast milk sweet. That's so babies would be encouraged to drink up the nutritious fluid and help ensure their survival, but it also means we're programmed to crave sweet things. I wish it weren't true, but any kind of added sugar in any food isn't good for you. As occasional treats, yes. As daily treats, sugary foods are killers.

The glycemic index (GI) is a rating system that ranks carbs on a scale of 1 to 100. The higher the number, the more that particular food will increase your blood sugar. Knowing these numbers can help you plan your meals. Steel-cut oats have a low GI, while instant oats are high. A low-calorie food like watermelon has a surprisingly high score of 76. Baked goods made with white flour and sugar, rice and potatoes and pasta, are all high on the GI as well.

There are lots of sugars in the world. Most of them should be avoided since they have no positive influence on your day-to-day health. Here are a few sugars to know about and understand:

- Glucose is a sugar that is critical for life. It is the basic fuel we burn to stay alive. When you hear the term "blood sugar," think glucose, as you read in Chapter 2.

- Table (or refined) sugar, that ubiquitous sweetener we buy in 5-pound bags for cooking, is a molecule called sucrose. Sucrose is made up of a glucose molecule bonded to a fructose molecule. When we eat anything sweetened with table sugar, our bodies break the bond in sucrose and quickly release one glucose and one fructose molecule each into our bloodstream.

- Fructose is also known as fruit sugar. It is, as you might expect, the sweet we taste when we eat most fruits. The difference we taste between any two fruits, such as a mango and a banana, is due to the esters and polyphenols unique to each fruit. Fruit sugar is not what our body burns. To use the sweet in fruit, we need to alter the fructose into glucose. That process takes energy to carry out, so fructose is not as efficient as glucose. And since too much fruit tends to put our bowels into overdrive and give us diarrhea, we do not usually eat enough fruit to make us fat. But . . .

- To satisfy our never-ending demand for sweet stuff, food manufacturers figured out how to concentrate the fructose from corn into high-fructose corn syrup, which is added to soda, candy, baked goods, and thousands of other foods. Even some brands of canned fruit and applesauce (What? Apples aren't sweet enough?), ketchup, barbecue sauce, salad dressing, and peanut butter have fructose added. Our bodies don't know what to do with such a giant load of fructose, so it's shunted directly to fat as quickly as your metabolism can manage.

- Honey is a massively complex mixture of glucose, phenols, polyphenols, glycols, and even a few peptides and proteins. Honey heals wounds and kills bacteria. It feeds bees and tastes great to every mammal on earth. If you must sweeten your food, a teaspoon or two of honey is a good choice.

- Fake sugars, or non-sugar sweeteners (NSS), were once thought to be diet aids, since they have no or very low calories. Those commonly used are acesulfame K, aspartame, cyclamates, saccharin, sucralose, and stevia. In May 2023, the World Health Organization released guidelines urging people not to use fake sugars, as studies have shown that the "use of NSS does not confer any long-term benefit in reducing body fat in adults or children. Results of the review also suggest that there may be potential undesirable effects from long-term use of NSS, such as an increased risk of type 2 diabetes, cardiovascular diseases, and mortality in adults." The risk of type 2 diabetes increases since your pancreas can't differentiate between real and fake sugar, so you get an insulin spike with both.

7. The brighter the color, the better the nutrients.

Vibrant red, green, yellow, purple, and orange fruits and vegetables are all good for you. Their phytochemicals, or bioactive compounds, create the different colors and show you that they're high in the fiber and micronutrients (vitamins and minerals) your body needs. All berries are loaded with antioxidants, which makes them a "superfood."

When your parents told you to eat your fruits and vegetables, they weren't kidding!

8. Put vegetables and salads at the center of your plate, with smaller servings of protein, especially red meat.

While you need daily protein in your diet (see page 199), you don't need as much as you think or you've been led to believe, especially when it comes to red meat. Red meat is flavorful and high in protein, which is good. On the other hand, red meat tends to increase inflammation, which you know is a killer. Most red meat sold in the U.S. comes from cattle that are plumped up with grains (not the grasses they're meant to eat) and dosed with antibiotics and growth hormones, which you certainly do not want to ingest.

If you do eat beef, it's best to buy only organic, grass-fed, and grass-finished meat. The better the diet for the animals, the more nutrients you will consume. Grass-fed means that the cattle may be pastured, but still plumped up with feed before going to the slaughterhouse, while grass-fed and grass-finished means the animals fed only on grass for their entire lives.

What to Eat for Longevity

While you can't control your genetic makeup, you can control what you eat. All you need is to eat is the right amount of food to fuel your metabolism. When you eat fewer calories, you're training your body to do more with less. And when you eat fresh whole foods, you will:

- Feel fuller faster and eat fewer calories.
- Stay satisfied longer from your newfound friend, fiber.
- Naturally be in the right calorie range.
- Keep your glycemic load on the low side.

When fed fresh whole foods, your body eagerly absorbs the nutrients critical for optimal hormone production and puts them to work right away. You won't need to count calories or grams of carbohydrates or fats. Eating for longevity is not about scarcity. It's all about learning how to eat the right foods in the right amounts that taste great so you can maintain healthy habits for the rest of your life.

The Proportions You Want to See on Your Plate

Divide your plate into the following fractions:

- ½ non-starchy vegetables and fruit
- ¼ lean protein and healthy fat
- ¼ starchy vegetables and whole grains

Note: 1 serving of healthy fat = approximately ½ small avocado, 1 tablespoon olive oil, 4 ounces fatty fish, 10 nuts, 1 tablespoon nut butter, or 5 olives.

Breakfast

- 4 to 6 ounces protein
- 1 serving healthy fat
- 1 to 2 servings high-fiber, low-glycemic carbohydrates

Lunch and/or Dinner

- 4 to 6 ounces lean protein
- 2 cups or more non-starchy, vibrantly colored vegetables (the more the better!)
- 1 to 3 servings healthy fats
- 1 serving high-fiber, starchy carbohydrate

The Best Foods for Longevity

Add as many of these foods to your daily diet as possible.

Eat Your Fruits and Vegetables

Plant foods contain powerful phytochemicals, such as carotenoids, the antioxidants that help protect your body from the free radicals that can damage your cells.

Found in fruits and vegetables of every color, carotenoids may also help to prevent cancer, play a role in anti-aging, enhance the function of your immune system, and support your reproductive system. In most cases, you can get all the carotenoids you need from eating plenty of orange, red, yellow, and green fruits and vegetables.

Cruciferous and other vegetables with strong flavors may help combat cancers of the breast, lung, colon, liver, and cervix. These vegetables include arugula, bok choy, broccoli, Brussels sprouts, cabbage, cauliflower, collard greens, kale, kohlrabi, mustard greens, radishes, rutabaga, turnips, and watercress.

Fiber-Rich Foods (Give Those Beans and Legumes Some Love)

High on the list of fiber-ful foods are complex carbohydrate plant foods: vegetables, fruits, beans, whole grains, nuts, and seeds. The fiber content in veggies increases your body's ability to burn fat by up to 30 percent. Complex carbohydrates in canned or dried beans and other legumes, like lentils, help keep your blood sugar levels balanced throughout the day. In turn, this helps lower insulin levels while providing a steady, slow-burning source of energy to make you feel awake. They are the richest source of soluble fiber, which is a key to good blood sugar control, and contain resistant starch RS1, which rebuilds the intestinal lining and creates short-term fatty acids that fight inflammation, cancer, and unfriendly microorganisms in the gut.

Go Nuts for Nuts!

Nuts are full of nutrients, satisfying, and portable. Grabbing a small handful—no more than ¼ cup—of protein-rich nuts will keep you going strong. Their healthy monounsaturated fats help protect you from heart disease, diabetes, and inflammation.

Many people are reluctant to eat nuts because of their high fat content, but research has shown that people who eat nuts twice a week are less likely to gain weight than those who don't. Pine nuts are especially good at helping prevent hunger, since they initiate the release of the appetite-suppressing hormone cholecystokinin, although some people can get a bitter or metallic taste in their mouth that lasts for some time. Pine nuts are also expensive compared to others.

Not Seedy at All

Seeds contain resistant starch that helps reduce blood sugar and slow down insulin spikes after eating. Flax is a great source of omega-3 fatty acids, which prevent inflammation. Flax meal (finely crushed flax seeds) is usually added to smoothies, oatmeal, or some baked goods. Don't eat too much at once as that can cause diarrhea. Pumpkin seeds are not only a good source of omega-3 fatty acids, but also of zinc, a key component in testosterone production and prostate health.

Why Protein Is Important—But You Don't Need as Much as You Think

You need protein to build and repair those all-important muscles, and for other metabolic functions. Eating protein does two important things:

1. Proteins are the single most difficult foods for the body to digest and use. Protein molecules are larger and more complex than others, such as fiber. Proteins require multiple energy-consuming steps to break them down into their component amino acids for use in your metabolic process. For every 500 calories of protein, you'll use about 100 calories to digest and process.

2. Protein energy is also released slowly over a longer period of time than fats or carbohydrates, which means that you won't get as hungry as soon. Try to eat some protein with every meal. Protein, like fats, also does not cause the insulin spikes that carbs do.

The biggest trick in high-protein diets is avoiding the excess fats they often contain. (Yes, you, keto diet!) Animal fats are rich in omega-6 fatty acids that increase the inflammatory processes throughout your body. (Omega-3 fatty acids, on the other hand, are anti-inflammatory.)

In addition, seniors need twice as much protein at 60 as they did at 20. The 25-year-old has a lot more muscle to support, but older folks simply do not process meats as efficiently as they did in our youth. One reason is that we need hydrochloric acid in our stomachs to break down the meat, but as we age, we produce less of this vital digestive component.

The average older woman should eat 1.5 grams of protein per day for every kilo (2.2 pounds) of body weight, and the average man 25 percent more per kilo of weight. An 8-ounce steak has 50 grams of protein; a cup of cottage cheese has 25 grams; and an egg has 6 grams.

A woman weighing 150 pounds (68 kilos) needs to eat about 100 grams of protein daily. There are about 37 grams in 1 ounce, so 55 grams is just under 2 ounces. That's not very much, is it?

Wild Salmon and Other Fatty Fish

Wild salmon, mackerel, black cod, herring, striped bass, sardines, and anchovies are rich in omega-3s, as well as a source of selenium, which is critical to your thyroid function. Omega-3-rich fish can decrease depression, lessen PMS symptoms, suppress inflammation, and counteract the inflammation caused by the omega-6 fatty acids found in meat. Omega-3s in salmon and in fully pastured meats and organic eggs may also help manage blood sugar and fight obesity.

Fermented Foods

Since our ancestors didn't have refrigeration to preserve foods, they discovered how to ferment them. As a side effect, they were improving their diets by adding much-needed good bacteria to their gut microbiomes and improving their bodies' digestive abilities. According to the National Institutes of Health, "Fermented foods provide many health benefits such as antioxidant, anti-microbial, anti-fungal, anti-inflammatory, anti-diabetic, and anti-atherosclerotic activity."

Fermented foods include sauerkraut, kimchi, and pickles, which are also low in calories and high in fiber. Miso, kombucha, unsweetened kefir, plain unsweetened yogurt, and apple cider vinegar are other good choices.

Spice It Up

Capsaicin, the chemical in hot peppers that makes your mouth burn, scalp itch, and body sweat also boosts your metabolism by up to 25 percent for as long as three hours. It's also found in hot sauces and chili peppers, and it's good for your gut. The smaller the chili pepper, the hotter it will be.

My wife is from Chengdu, China, where they worship the chili pepper. I jokingly told her that her cooking got a lot better once my taste buds died from heat. When we go to a Thai restaurant, she says, "Bring it on!" and asks for extra chili powder on the side. She eats fiery foods and sauces without breaking a sweat, while I just gape in awe.

What to Drink

Hydration Needs

"You must drink eight cups of water a day or you'll pass out from dehydration!" Where did that advice come from?'

Not from me, that's for sure. Yes, you need to drink several cups of water every day, not including coffee or tea, depending where you are. Drink enough water so you don't feel thirsty in your environment. I was recently in Arizona, where the temperature was 95°F and the humidity was close to zero every day, I was chugging water by the gallon trying to stay hydrated. My lips were still chapped a week later. That doesn't happen in rainy Seattle!

The best way to gauge if you're drinking enough water is to look at the color of your urine. If your urine is dark yellow, drink more water. If you're peeing every hour, you need to see a doctor. Stop guzzling from those overpriced and overhyped designer water bottles that create tons of plastic and damage the environment. I recommend that you always filter your drinking water no matter where you live by using a water filter pitcher or installing a water filter faucet.

Coffee and Tea Time

I love my morning jolt of caffeine—a three- or four-ounce black espresso before my morning workout and one cappuccino after my breakfast. I might have an additional half-cup of coffee in the office. Then I switch to caffeine-free peach green tea for the rest of the day.

Small amounts of caffeine have well-proven health benefits. It boosts your metabolic rate and suppresses your appetite. The catechins in coffee and tea tend to suppress fat production, can help lower your risk and growth of many cancers. and produce alertness by reducing levels of a molecule called adenosine. Adenosine tends to promote better sleep and reduce the inflammation that can lead to heart disease, diabetes, and organ damage.

That's the good news. The bad news is that too much caffeine triggers your stress response, raising cortisol and consequently insulin levels as well as your blood pressure. It also disturbs sleep.

The FDA recommends drinking no more than 400 mg of caffeine every day. That's about 20 ounces of black coffee, 40 ounces of black tea, or 110 ounces of green tea. I tell my patients to switch from their morning coffee or black tea to caffeine-free herbal or green teas if they want more hot or cold drinks during the rest of the day.

Green tea is the closest thing to a metabolism-jolting potion you can find. It contains a plant compound that promotes fat burning. In one study, people who consumed three to five cups a day for 12 weeks decreased their body weight by 4.6 percent and burned an extra 50 calories a day. In addition, green tea contains a compound called ECGC (epigallocatechin gallate), which has been shown to inhibit the growth of a wide variety of cancers.

The Worst Foods for Longevity

Packaged, Refined Foods

Eating refined foods is like trying to keep a bonfire going with toilet paper. Your body (the bonfire) quickly consumes the refined foods (the toilet paper), but does not get enough sustenance to keep itself fueled for long. After a brief boost, you will need to eat more refined foods just to keep going even as you wonder why you're so hungry after you just ate a huge bagel with a big schmear of cream cheese.

During the process of refining foods, nutrients are lost and valuable fiber is removed. What's left is a bland, nutrient-poor, calorie-rich shell of the original food. Many refined foods are so far from their original forms nutritionally that synthetic nutrients and flavorings like sugar and salt are added to give the foods some phony flavor. Your body processes refined foods differently than it does whole foods. For example, take a handful of whole grains like oats and a handful of white flour. Let each one sift through your fingers. What do you notice? The whole grains go through slowly, while the white flour runs through like water.

Additives like artificial sweeteners, emulsifiers, and other chemicals like preservatives can affect the microbiome in your gut because they aren't recognized as "real" foods. High-fructose corn syrup will screw up your blood sugar. Ditto the cheap and longer shelf-life trans fats (liquid oils processed into solid fats) that affect cholesterol levels and can lead to heart attacks, strokes, and diabetes.

Be a smart consumer. Read the labels. If you see a long list of sugars (especially high-fructose corn syrup), fats (especially trans fats), and additives, preservatives, and chemicals you can't pronounce, you're wasting your money on junk food that often costs far more than fresh, whole foods and that can wreck your health.

Never Food Shop on an Empty Stomach

Never go grocery shopping when you're hungry. Make a list of what you need and stick to it. Fill your cart with fresh foods. Canned or frozen fruits are okay as long as no sugar or other ingredients are added. Don't impulse buy because the items are inevitably going to be high-fat, loaded with sugars, and high in calories. If you don't have junk food in the house, you can't eat it!

What Not to Drink

Don't Drink Your Calories!

Many of my patients work hard to improve what they eat, but they don't realize what's actually contained in many beverages they consume. Smoothies, especially when made from fresh veggies, can be healthy and satisfying. But many of those sold in smoothie shops are sugar-dense calorie bombs. While a cup of black coffee has no calories, a latte or cappuccino can range from 100 to 500+ calories, thanks to the milk and sugar added—and it will send your blood sugar skyrocketing. An eight-ounce glass of orange juice contains about 100 calories (and little fiber), while a fresh orange contains half the caloric amount and is full of fiber. It's easier to drink a lot of juice than to eat whole pieces of fruit!

Banishing Booze

There's nothing wrong with enjoying an occasional glass of wine, but there aren't any health benefits from drinking alcohol regularly. The beneficial component found in red wine (and grape juice) is resveratrol, a powerful phytochemical that helps fight viruses, diabetes, heart disease, and inflammation. The problem is that a five-ounce glass of red wine contains 0.03 to1.07 mg of resveratrol, and the average daily dose in a recommended supplement is 100 to 1,000 mg.

In addition, alcohol is a toxin that increases estrogen in your bloodstream, promotes fat storage, and decreases muscle growth. As soon as you have a drink, your body gobbles up all the glycogen in your liver, making you hungry, and the sudden intake of alcohol makes you tipsy, which reduces inhibitions. If you drink too much alcohol you are likely to eat more food and drink even more. You also burn less fat, and it burns more slowly than normal.

No amount of alcohol is good for you. If you do want a drink, treat it as you would a slice of cheesecake—an occasional indulgence.

Soda/Jerks

Except for club soda or seltzer, no carbonated soda is good for you. Even diet soda. Here's the problem: It's not the sugar; it's the sweet. Whenever you drink anything that tastes sweet, your metabolism shifts because your body thinks there are high calories coming in and braces itself to process them all. You'll get an insulin and blood sugar spike, and the excess will, as you now know, be stored as fat. Many sodas also contain caffeine as well as ascorbic, carbonic, and phosphoric acids to make the carbonation. They leach calcium from your bones and all that acid can harm your teeth.

If you like to drink something with fizz in it, flavored club sodas contain no sugar. Or, add a few citrus fruit slices to your plain water or club soda and enjoy.

It's Not That Hard to Cook!

I call myself a survival cook. If you eat what I cook, you will survive. But I make no promises beyond that!

That said, shopping for and cooking your own food is the only way to control exactly what ingredients you're eating. Buying fresh food is going to be much more economical than eating out or depending on junk food. A five-*pound* bag of potatoes costs the same (or less) as a five-*ounce* bag of potato chips!

Add some spice to your life (literally) by experimenting with new foods and new recipes. There are millions of recipes online and countless YouTube tutorials if you want some guidance. Have a friend or friends over to keep you company (and help you) in the kitchen.

If you don't like what you bought, put any vegetables in a stockpot and add water to make a broth and freeze it in small portions. When I was a starving student, we kept a stockpot on low heat on the stove when we were home. While we couldn't afford much meat, the butcher always had some inexpensive bones that we added, along with some barley, beans, and odds and ends of veggies. By the end of the week, we had a great stew that was delicious, nutritious, satisfying, and dirt cheap.

Since you won't be spending money on expensive restaurant meals or takeout food, you will be able to buy better-quality food. You deserve the best and that means the best foods you can afford.

How My Patient Richard Tonelli Eats

Remember 86-year-old Richard from Chapter 6? Here's his meal routine:

My philosophy of eating is like Dr. Mixon's: I eat two healthy meals a day: a large breakfast at 7 a.m. and a big lunch around 1 p.m. I try to stop eating after 5 p.m.

Breakfast

Breakfast often consists of one cup of coffee, three hard-boiled eggs, a variety of unsalted nuts, one banana, blueberries, raspberries, two dates, ¼ apple, and other fruits. I also take fiber and protein/collagen powders and several supplements.

Lunch

Lunch starts with the leanest red meat, fish (mostly salmon), or chicken. Most of my meat comes from Costco. I cook it, divide into serving portions, place in ziplock bags, and freeze. I like having a choice of just-need-heating main courses for lunch. I wrap a sweet potato or a few Yukon gold potatoes in wet paper towels and microwave until they're done. Then I add butter and salt to the hot potatoes. While the potatoes are cooking, I steam some vegetables: Brussels sprouts, green beans, asparagus, broccoli, and/or beets. I make a large salad with greens, onions, tomatoes, radishes, Kalamata olives, and avocado, and toss everything with salt, pepper, olive oil, and balsamic vinegar.

Snacks

My occasional snacks are popcorn or a square of dark chocolate. I rarely eat dessert.

Recommended Supplements for Weight Management

Refer to Chapter 5 for more details. Discuss the proper doses for your needs as well as any potential contraindications with your doctor before taking any new supplements.

Fiber Number one on the list is a supplement such as FiberCon or Metamucil—unless you are already eating a diet high in fiber-rich foods. Take it daily, before you eat. Other fiber supplements will also work; it's a matter of which one your gut will tolerate. (Some people can't tolerate psyllium, for example.) Start with a very low dose (maybe half of the recommended dose) and increase gradually as you will produce gas until the bacteria in your gut adjust. If you become very gassy or bloated, then reduce the amount by at least half. Keep Gas-X on hand as it does help minimize gas. Once your gut gets used to the new fiber, usually over several weeks, your bacteria will handle fiber far more efficiently and the gas will go away.

Omega-3 Fatty Acids Fish oil capsules of 1.8 grams of EPA a day have been shown to increase insulin sensitivity, which is important for people who have become insulin resistant.

Metformin or Berberine Prescription-only Metformin as well as berberine help with blood sugar regulation.

MultiVitamin/Mineral If you're eating a lot less food, you might be vitamin or mineral deficient. A basic vitamin/mineral supplement will help. If you're concerned, have your blood drawn to check your micronutrient levels so you don't take more supplements than you need.

Chapter 9
Smarter

Losing cognitive function is one of the things that frightens us as we get older. Sure, we all laugh at those senior moments. You know, you walk into a room, stand there, and wonder, *Why did I come in here? What am I looking for?* Or, you might run into someone you've known for years and can't remember their name. Those are small signs that you have age-related cognitive decline. Your brain is not working as well as it used to. You've lost neurons (brain cells). You've lost connections between neurons. You start to panic.

That's where Rule #8 comes in: If the brain doesn't work, the rest doesn't matter.

The brain is a delicate structure and it does not grow very fast. Skin cells in young people turn over every two or three weeks. Ten percent of your bone is replaced every year. Brain neurons live for years before they're turned over. But when you kill brain cells, or they just naturally die at the end of their life span, replacing them is a slow, painstaking process. Frankly, most of us are not strong enough or fit enough, or don't exercise enough or provide ourselves with the proper nutrition we need, to grow enough new brain tissue. What you lose, you lose. The trick is to not lose those brain cells in the first place.

Just as our muscles shrink over time, so do our brains. That's a natural function that occurs in every human being. Fortunately, there are easy and inexpensive ways to help you grow back some of your brain and maintain its function as you age.

Your Brain Does Not Age Like Fine Wine

Testing for Cognitive Decline

Brain function decline is almost never smooth or predictable over every cognitive domain, so cognitive testing can be very useful. When we check brain function at our clinics, we look at six different areas of cognition: short-term memory processing, long-term memory processing, speed of processing, executive functions (such as decision-making skills), motor skills, and spatial orientation and recognition.

Computerized tests can process enormous amounts of information, far more than any one person can. It's best to have your physician evaluate your results, as people grading their own tests tend to upgrade themselves significantly. Let's face it, most of us are notoriously bad at evaluating ourselves. (Eight out of ten Americans think they look younger than their age!) Our clinics use a 30-minute online test, the Cambridge Brain Function study. (One is from Cambridge, U.K., and one is from Cambridge, Canada; I prefer the Canadian test.) It uses different parameters to tell you where you are compared to other people your age and gender. Of course, that's a rough number to start with because a PhD astrophysicist is probably going to begin with a much higher cognitive function than a high school dropout. But if the PhD astrophysicist is functioning at only the median level for the population in his age group, he's likely lost a lot of his brain function and needs further evaluation.

A fair bit of this initial evaluation will be based on the doctor's evaluation. The critical point comes when the test is repeated a year later, and the previous year's results are compared to the most recent ones. That is what we're looking for: Are you improving or holding your own? If you are declining, then we need to increase intensity of your program and follow you closely.

Accelerating Brain Shrinkage

No one wants brain shrinkage, but there are several things guaranteed to speed up the process:

- Genetic factors. A family history of neurological disorders such as Alzheimer's disease, or genetic disorders such as Huntington's disease.
- Alcohol, heavy smoking, chronic drug use, and other toxins. The easiest and quickest way to kill your brain cells is to starve them of oxygen. Any toxin will do that, especially alcohol, the most common toxin in America. The only reason our bodies can tolerate grain alcohol (ethyl alcohol) is because we've evolved to handle the small amounts of it produced in our guts when the carbohydrates in our diets are fermented by the yeast and bacteria in our microbiome. Whenever you drink alcohol, it is processed in the liver, and the liver tries to get rid of it before it can reach the brain. You know your liver hasn't gotten rid of enough alcohol when you wake up with a hangover or can't remember what you did after drinking too much or taking certain drugs.
- Sedentary lifestyle, with weakening muscles and/or sarcopenia.
- A diet high in carbohydrates and sugar. A simple blood test measures the level of hemoglobin A1C, which tells us what percentage of your red blood cells have been damaged by glucose. As your average blood sugar rises, the rate of brain shrinkage increases, faster and faster—more than twice as fast, in fact. (This doesn't even factor in the damage that can be done by diabetes.)

Brain Shrinkage and Women

Here's another difference between women and men. When a man gets married, he's signing on for several different women in his life. Let me explain:

- He starts off with a woman in her mating and dating mode; Mother Nature has made sure she does everything possible to demonstrate her sexual appeal and prowess to mate.

- After they get married, that mating/dating/sexual instinct phase extinguishes itself over the next year or so because the woman has already mated. This is the underlying biology for the old saw that sexual passion begins with adolescence and ends with marriage.

- When the woman has a baby, she has no control over the biological imperative to restructure her brain. It literally changes shape. First it grows a bit, and then it remodels its micro-circuitry so that the husband is no longer the central focus of her life; the baby is. (This may be one reason some men have trouble adjusting to that new reality, where they are no longer the center of attention.) Mommy brain is a real thing. As the cognitive executive functions of a mother's brain shrink, the nurturing, supportive parts of her brain increase. The original size and micro-circuitry are never the same again. When the brain swells, shrinks, and then regrows, things can go wrong. This is that dangerous period when a woman may develop post-partum depression or, in rare situations, overt psychosis.

- When a woman hits menopause, estrogen levels drop, progesterone levels fall even further, testosterone levels crater, inflammation increases, and neurons start to die faster. Women tend to maintain verbal skills far longer than men do, but with less estrogen, they become worse at verbal processing. Since women's brains are smaller in size than men's, they tend to lose functionality a little faster. With less brain tissue to begin with women can afford to lose less. (On the other hand, men have more strokes and kill more of their brain with vascular issues.) If we replace their hormones, we can often protect the brains of both men and women.

Keeping Your Brain Healthy

You can undo the damage, or at least some of it, depending on how badly the brain is damaged. Those who are proactive about this starting at age 40 or 50, when they haven't lost a lot of brain tissue, can improve. After that, you need to try to stop, or at least slow, any future loss.

Decrease Inflammation

The most important thing you can do is decrease inflammation. This will lower your risk of dementia (as well as your cholesterol levels and risk of diabetes, heart attacks, and strokes—see Chapter 3 for a refresher).

Get That Blood Flowing

The other thing you need to do is maintain or even increase the blood flow to your brain. If your blood pressure is at the high end of normal or higher, use a vasodilator medication such as an ACE inhibitor or an ACE receptor blocker. Use supplements that increase nitric oxide production such as citrulline, or Neo40. Foods like beets help. Regular exercise develops collateral flow to the brain regions. Erectile dysfunction drugs all increase blood flow to the brain as well as to the genitals, which is why I put most of my patients, male and female, on them.

Take Your B Vitamins

Taking a multi-B vitamin supplement every day decreases brain shrinkage.

Move It, Move It, Move It to Make Your Muscles Stronger

The more muscle you have and the more intensely and frequently that muscle is used, the more you kick out a chemical growth trigger, BDNF (brain-derived neurotrophic factor), which encourages brain tissue growth and heals and repairs damage to the brain.

The problem, as I've said, is that as you get older, you become tired so you don't always feel like exercising. If your joints hurt, you don't want to stress them because that's painful, so you sit down and rest instead. It becomes a vicious negative destructive cycle. This is why you need to get rid of the inflammation and the pain, and increase your hormones so your brain says, *Damn, I feel good. I think I'm going for a walk. Or maybe I'll swim laps. I know—I'll have a jog on the treadmill.* And you do it!

Here is a reminder of the importance of working muscle and good supplementation. A professional writer came to the clinic because he noticed that his facility for finding the right words was declining. He was concerned that his writing days might be over because of what he called his "brain fog." He sat for hours staring at his computer screen, unable to come up with the correct words to describe what he had in mind. We were able to help get him out of his rut with a daily exercise routine and supplements to improved his cognition. He lost 25 pounds and returned eight of his major hormone levels back to a young man's values. After six months on the program, he is stronger, faster, leaner, smarter, and back to writing. He claims that his facility with language is as good as it ever was. I do not know about sexier in his case. But he is a very happy patient.

Manage Your Blood Sugar, Which Means Lose Weight

As you read in Chapter 3, as glucose is circulating throughout your body, it's damaging every tissue it touches, including the red blood cells in your bloodstream. The higher your average sugar, the more red blood cells have been damaged, and this affects your brain shrinkage.

The normal range for hemoglobin A1C is 4.4 to 5.6 percent of the red blood cells.

- If your A1C is 4.4 to 5.2, you're in the bottom half of the normal range. This is just where we want you to be. At the target number of 5.2 and below, you are losing about 0.25 percent of your brain tissue each year, which happens to everyone as they age.

- If your A1C is 5.7, you are pre-diabetic. You are increasing the rate of your brain volume loss by 50 percent to losing about 0.375 percent of your brain volume each year. This means that about 0.5 percent of your brain is shrinking every year, twice the baseline rate of 0.25 percent with that lower the rate to 0.2 percent and below.
- By the time you're at 5.9, you've more than doubled the rate of brain loss. And your brain is shrinking even faster. You are now losing 0.5 percent of your brain volume every year. And as your A1C continues to rise, so does the rate at which you lose brain volume. This is a big part of why dementia is more common in diabetics, who have almost three times the risk of dementia than non-diabetics.
- Bear in mind that most doctors who are treating diabetics will tell them that they're fine even if their A1C is 7.5 because it's within the "normal" range. They're not fine. At 7.5, your brain is rotting away.

As an aside, something unexpected about the keto diet is that those who go on it are eating low carbs and fewer calories, yet they feel great. Their emotional state improves because their brain has shifted from burning sugar to burning ketone bodies, which allows them to feed their brains more efficiently. (The problem with the keto diet is that it's high in fat and low in fiber, as you know, so I don't recommend it for long-term weight control.)

Increase Hormone Levels

Your anabolic sex hormones are neurotransmitters that alter how you feel. Most doctors don't understand the neurologic biochemistry of estrogen, testosterone, progesterone, and pregnenolone and how they are mood modulators. All of these hormones are critical for brain function and emotional regulation yet are rarely prescribed for these conditions.

For more, see the section on Hormones and Your Brain on page 218 in Chapter 9.

Increase Your Omega-3 Intake

Fats make up the primary components for brain tissue. Most of the brain fat is comprised of the omega fats DHA and EPA, especially your neurons. This is part of why omega-3 fats are critically important to maintain and repair brain tissue and peripheral nerves.

Fats are basically oils that are solid at room temperature. Whether plant or animal, nearly every living thing makes oils as an inevitable component of living tissues. You should ingest at least two tablespoons of a good fat every day—fish or nut oils, extra-virgin olive oil, avocado oil, sunflower oil—as they are essential to keep our brains functioning. Avoid partially hydrogenated transfats such as shortening and margarine. Eating too much bad fat increases the inflammation that kills brain tissue.

Use It or Lose It

Like everything else in your body, you want to use it or lose it. I used to have dozens of phone numbers in my head. And now . . . our smartphones have made us dumb! I don't even know my wife's number. But I'm great at touching her name on the screen and the call goes right through!

You've probably heard the old myth that we use only a small part of our brain. That's not true. Your entire brain is always active, processing information during the day, and dreaming at night. That doesn't mean your brain isn't lazy. When your brain can get a hack to be lazy, your brain will always take the hack. So you want to practice as many different modalities of learning as you can.

Do Brain Exercises Work?

Brain exercises tend to improve only the area of the brain that you're exercising. You'll get better at a particular task if you do it regularly, but you won't necessarily improve other cognitive skills. If you're learning a new language, or memorizing Shakespeare or the phone numbers you've forgotten, for example, you become good at memorization, but that it won't help you follow a schematic. Puzzle solving helps with executive function. A crossword puzzle fanatic with dementia might not recognize family members, but he might still be able to do crossword puzzles.

I don't do specific memory tests or skills, but I spend several hours every day reading and evaluating medical journal articles. I talk to other doctors. I teach my physicians. I try to wrangle visits with the top researchers around the world. I talk to them on the phone and email them, and when possible, I fly to their centers to discuss their research and how it pertains to longevity. I do everything I can to stay cognitively engaged almost every waking hour.

You want to be cognitively engaged in whichever way fits into your life every day as well. To strive for more brain power, try to learn something new outside of your wheelhouse. Make it something that challenges you intellectually and/or physically and that interests you enough to do daily.

When I was single, I memorized romantic poems because the women I was dating liked them. Some people learn to code. If you follow a religious tradition, learn your scripture. Study topics along with your kids. Play card games with your friends. If you were challenged by math in school, you know what? Even at 60 you can get yourself a basic algebra book and tackle it. (I bring this up because my daughter asks me for help with her math homework, and I don't have a clue. I go on YouTube for tutorials . . . and I still don't have a clue! But it is helping me with numbers. Besides, falling down that YouTube rabbit hole can lead you to all kinds of fascinating topics to keep your brain engaged.)

What can help even more is to do an activity that utilizes different parts of your brain that you haven't typically used—learning to sing or play a new instrument, or taking dance classes or any kind of movement class that involves repetition. This will improve your kinesthetic memory. Studies of professional dancers have shown that they have strong neural connectivity in their general motor learning network, which will help them with balance and coordination as they get older.

Your Brain and Your Balance

Speaking of balance and coordination, this is an area where old folks usually lose capacity, as you learned already. My mother's panicked call reminds me of the now-infamous "I've fallen and I can't get up," which usually has multiple components: Falling often is triggered in part by the loss of balance and less active proprioceptors in our joints and extremities, as you read in Chapter 7. In addition, central balance from the brainstem starts to fade as we age. And vision and middle ear balance mechanisms are slowly going bad.

Add to that the loss of strength in both your extremities and central core muscles, and you are setting yourself up for falling. Even if you don't fracture a bone in a fall, you might have trouble getting up. A 70-plus-year-old on the floor has a lot more trouble bouncing to his feet than a 10-year-old. Together, all of these issues are part of the problem. What do we do about them?

Strength training and developing flexibility are a big part of improving balance, as you read in Chapter 7. Some of you might be saying to yourself, "I thought this section was on cognition, not muscle." Guess what? Brain function and practice are a big part of what we are addressing here. If you do not practice something you lose the skill set. Most 70-year-olds don't get down on the floor to do yoga or stretching exercises, so they have no practice in the process of getting up. The muscles, nerves, and central brain functions needed for the job have atrophied from lack of use.

The dichotomy between brain and body is an error. The brain is a part of the body. Those nerves in control that run from the brain down the spinal cord and into our muscles are simply an extension of the brain! Brain function, muscle function, and balance are all a part of the same issue: a body that has allowed some of its important functions to atrophy through disuse. You need to fix that!

Do the exercise in the sidebar on the next page, and then go back to Chapter 7 and do the other balance exercises faithfully. Doing these exercises for a few minutes every day can make an enormous difference in your balance and coordination. Any kind of exercise that involves balance, such as squats, push-ups, or side-to-side moves, will help. Do planks to strengthen your core muscle. If you stopped exercising, get back to doing the physically difficult things you quit doing a long time ago, and do some of them every day before you find yourself helpless on the floor.

Rebuild the capacity to think, to learn, to move, and to feel confident with your balance. They are all critical parts of lifelong health.

A Balance Training Move for Your Brain and Body

Stand near a wall or next to a sturdy couch or chair. (This is to catch you or provide a security aid if needed.) Close your eyes and raise your left foot off the floor so you're standing only on your right leg. Bend your left knee and then straighten it back up. Do this a few times and repeat with the other leg. To make it more challenging, cross your hands over your chest while doing it. If you feel like you're losing your balance, put your leg down and use the couch or chair for support until you feel secure on the ground again. If this is too much for you, simply bend both knees at the same time and then straighten your legs. Do as many as you can without strain or pain.

Hormones and Your Brain

Hormones are needed in adequate doses to stave off brain loss and inflammation. When estrogen, progesterone, and testosterone levels plummet, drive, ambition, self-confidence, and stress tolerance plummet with them—while fears and anxieties increase. Time for a re-think!

Estrogen and Your Brain

Estradiol, the primary human estrogen, is a potent anti-inflammatory and is important for maintaining a woman's brain size during and after menopause. It also improves verbal skills while lowering the risk of dementia, heart attacks, and depression. When you start taking estrogen for other conditions, you should notice that you're having fewer cognitive issues and your moods will likely improve.

Too many women in perimenopause or menopause are automatically prescribed antidepressants when they are having mood swings, depression symptoms, or anxiety. Here is a news flash for the psychiatric community: Menopause is not a serotonin deficiency! It is a poly-hormonal deficit. Women need the primary human psychoactive steroid, testosterone. They also need both estrogens and real, human-type, bio-identical progesterone—not a synthetic version. If a doctor thinks a woman might be depressed, she needs her hormones checked immediately. And the doctor should be looking at testosterone as the primary hormone deficiency in depressed women and men. Testosterone provides emotional security, self-confidence, stress tolerance, and enthusiasm, in addition to libido. Men and women both lose these mental characteristics as testosterone and DHEA levels wane. Estrogen is critical for verbal processing, and emotional stability. But the big hit in estrogen loss is rising systemic brain inflammation, which is one of the major triggers of depression. Every NSAID (nonsteroidal anti-inflammatory drug) pill on the market, such as ibuprofen and ketoprofen (prescribed for arthritis), is an antidepressant. The problem with NSAIDS as antidepressants is that they're so tough on the GI tract, liver, and heart that you can't take them long-term. (By the way, the anti-inflammatory effect of estrogen also protects your heart and your joints from damage.)

Of course, clinical depression needs to be addressed by investigating the root causes as scrupulously as possible before prescription mental health meds are suggested. Medication may be necessary if you have a serious condition or an acute episode, but one of the biggest problems with many antidepressants and anti-psychotics is that they cause weight gain, so increased insulin resistance can result. This can be a double whammy for women who may not need these meds yet are putting on pounds that make them feel worse. Psychoactive drugs often interfere with both sex drive and emotional satisfaction with intimacy. They can often introduce more problems than benefits if the diagnosis is inaccurate.

For men, estrogen is also important. We measure estrogen every time we do a lab panel and find that we seldom need to prescribe it. Men make their estrogen not in their nonexistent ovaries, but in their fat cells. They also make it out of testosterone. When we raise a man's testosterone, the estrogen he needs will increase automatically. Occasionally, a man comes to us whose body fat is so low he cannot convert testosterone to estrogen, but that is rare. If needed, men can use both estradiol and testosterone creams to get to the healthy levels they need. Just as in women, the estradiol is a potent anti-inflammatory. It also improves a man's verbal skills and word recall.

Thyroid Hormones and Your Brain

Your T3 and T4 are important brain hormones, regulating not only your physical energy but emotional and cognitive energy. If your thyroid function is low, your brain slows down; you get brain fog, you feel tired, you're lethargic, and you can't get out the door to exercise.

Get your levels checked and discuss your options with your doctor if you're on the low end of "normal." Refer to page 115 in Chapter 4 for more information about TSH results. The ideal TSH range is between 0.8 and 1.5. At this range, most people feel far more energetic and awake than they do at the higher ranges of normal TSH.

Dementia and Neurological Decline

The fear of dementia is palpable and understandable. Being alive, yet not yourself, is not how anyone wants to spend their later years, especially knowing the enormous toll dementia and Alzheimer's disease takes on loved ones. Dementia is on the rise as well, most notably since we're living longer. When nearly everybody died young, dementia was not an issue.

With cognitive deficits, you often don't recognize you have them. You can make bad decisions and not know you're making them. That's why with early onset Alzheimer's, everyone around the person sees the decline and may be telling them, yet the sufferer is outraged at the idea, sometimes insisting in full paranoia that there are plots against them since they are certain they're perfectly fine. They cannot perceive how their brain function is deteriorating. And the worst thing about this is that their previous brain function will never return. It just gets worse and worse.

There are four different kinds of dementia:

- Genetic dementias, such frontotemporal dementia and Alzheimer's disease. As you read in Chapter 3, those with the APO epsilon 4 gene from both parents have a 50/50 chance of showing signs of dementia by age 60. People focus on the 50 percent who will develop dementia, not the 50 percent who don't. They've all got the same genome—showing that the genome is propensity, not destiny. The 50 percent who didn't develop the dementia likely had a lifestyle that protected them. If you have a family history of dementia, get a genetic screening test. You should know if you're at risk.

- Toxic dementia is due to infections or exposure to heavy metals, pesticides, herbicides, and/or toxins that damage the brain. There are tests that can identify levels of these substances in your bloodstream. Once you are diagnosed and get the offending agents out of your body, you should improve or not worsen.

- Vascular dementia refers to having hundreds of micro-strokes causing what are called lacuna, which resemble little moons on an MRI. These mini strokes kill off tiny pieces of the brain, no one of these strokes is enough to impair your function. But over time, if you keep having them, the damage adds up and your cognition goes to hell.

- Age-related cognitive decline is simply losing grey matter as we age, which happens to most people. It is considered normal, and it usually starts with a falling-off in creativity and short-term memory. When problems arise, older people tend to look at how the problems were solved in their youth as opposed to looking for creative answers to the current problem.

The good news is that strong muscles and maintenance of robust hormone levels, coupled with an active physical and mental lifestyle, can avert most of the age-related cognitive decline. These are the action steps you should take to decrease inflammation and stave off dementia:

- Get plenty of antioxidants in your diet. Eat lots and lots of vibrantly colored fresh vegetables.

- Make sure you have plenty of fiber in your diet. If you have a less-than-ideal fiber-rich diet, take a fiber supplement every day.

- Keep your blood sugar as low as possible.
- Exercise regularly. Not just walking but developing muscle with strength training and using that muscle regularly. Being a weekend warrior isn't enough!
- Have a physician who is an expert in multi-hormone replacement restore as many of your endocrine-support hormones to youthful levels as possible.
- If you think there are issues or something is not quite right, get evaluated by a neurologist as soon as possible. Remember, if the brain doesn't work, the rest doesn't matter. Most neurologists, like other physicians, are looking for "normal," not "optimal" function. "Normal" is age-related decline! Do not accept the statement, "You are perfectly normal *for your age.*" That should never be your goal. You want to be evaluated using a young person as your standard of achievement.

Gerontologists are expert in juggling the multiple medications usually prescribed to older people as their bodies are progressively falling apart. They are not anti-aging/longevity doctors, so their focus is different.

Recommended Supplements for Brain Power

Refer to Chapter 5 for more details. Discuss the proper doses for your needs as well as any potential contraindications with your doctor before taking any new supplements.

Acetyl-L-carnitine Made from L-carnitine in your body, it doesn't reverse dementia, but peer-reviewed studies show that it can slow the rate at which you lose your ability to process information. On the other hand, age-related cognitive decline, which is less severe than overt dementia, has been shown to be improved to a modest degree in several studies. I take it, even though I show no evidence of decline at 76 years of age, other than the occasional lapse while searching for a specific word. I figure, if it improves mild, age-related decline, I might as well keep it in my system to see if I can avoid as much decline as possible.

Antioxidants, such as vitamins C and E. These can help protect neurons from oxidative damage. Take vitamin C and vitamin E together. Vitamin C recycles the vitamin E and recharges it after it's used, so you can absorb more of it.

B Vitamins Any brand of a comprehensive B supplement will do. Taking these vitamins is one of the easiest and least expensive ways to protect your brain from shrinking.

Resveratrol This phytonutrient can improve blood flow to the brain and is also a potent anti-inflammatory agent that inhibits the formation of senescent cells. Only a small portion of what you swallow will be absorbed, so you need a high dose. I take three 350 mg capsules every day. My wife, who is half my size, takes two 350 mg caps daily.

Chapter 10
Sexier

My goal with this book is to help people who are aging become stronger, faster, leaner, smarter, and sexier. Sexier comes last on the list, but it certainly isn't the least when it comes to achieving longevity goals. What you can do to be a more sexual human being is also what you do to be a healthier, stronger, faster, leaner, smarter, and happier human being. If your desire to be sexy and to want sex is fading, it's a sign that something is wrong. As a result, a large percentage of our senior population is celibate, whether due to social circumstances, lowered libido, or medical conditions or diseases that affect sexual performance.

Everything you've read in this book so far is meant to help set you up for a robust and passionate romantic life. I'm fed up with our society making us feel that loss of libido is inevitable as we get older and that nothing can be done about it once we reach our 50s, 60s, and beyond. If you are a vigorous, sexually active senior, you're often considered outside the norm when you shouldn't be.

Of course, it is always easier to prevent problems than to fix them. Restoring or increasing libido without improving the ability to function (because of erectile dysfunction for men or vaginal pain for women) is not a good thing. If you want to have sex but can't, that needs to be rectified.

About Sexual Dysfunction

For most of human history, few people lived to the age of 50. Men were designed to be able to impregnate as many women as they could have sex with throughout their natural life spans. But Mother Nature knew that childbearing becomes more dangerous as women get older and the chances of genetic defects increase as well. She made certain that women would be fertile and men would be fully functional up to a certain age. That's why women become infertile after menopause and 50 percent of men over the age of 50 have some level of erectile dysfunction.

As hormone production declines, it doesn't just affect your brain, muscles, bones, and organs. It also affects how you feel and how well you function physically and sexually.

Erectile Dysfunction in Men

Many men don't think they have erectile dysfunction until they can't have an erection, but the problem starts when their erections are less strong. Tumescence (the readiness for sexual activity) becomes less profound, often starting when men are in their late 30s or early 40s, but if they can achieve orgasm, they consider themselves okay.

This is a generalized healthcare issue with men that I refer to as the Rambo complex. We men have the tendency to equate illness with weakness, which leads to denial. Erectile dysfunction is such an emotionally charged area that most men will admit it exists only when the problem becomes so bad that we can no longer function.

The good news is that the problem can often be corrected, at least to a degree. The earlier the intervention, the better the results of our treatment. I recommend starting treatment as soon as there is any decline in the firmness or duration of a man's erection. At that point, only simple lifestyle interventions like weight loss and exercise may be necessary. Most men don't know that there is a direct correlation between abdominal girth and erectile function. The bigger your belly, the less sexually potent you are likely to be. That same rule applies to heart disease: Erectile dysfunction and cardiac events are tied to disorders of the arteries. When you have erectile dysfunction, your risk of dying from cardiac disease or developing dementia goes up dramatically.

Vaginal Atrophy in Women

As estrogen levels decline, the vagina undergoes changes; it starts to atrophy. The tissues of the vaginal wall become thinner. With less natural lubrication, the vagina becomes drier and there is a loss of elasticity. The vagina no long stretches to accommodate intercourse, and there can be inflammation within the vaginal walls. This may lead to urinary symptoms and make having sex extremely painful or even impossible.

Raising estrogen, progesterone, and testosterone levels is the first step to improving vaginal health. A bioidentical hormone cream can be applied to any part of the body, and suppositories can be inserted vaginally. The more of the skin's surface, the thinner the skin, and the richer the blood supply, the better the response. I encourage women to apply their testosterone on their clitoris, because the mucus membranes in the vulva absorb any of the sex hormones 12 times more efficiently than on skin elsewhere on the body. A testosterone cream will also increase lubrication, as it will be converted to estradiol by the fat in the tissues and the clitoris will enlarge a bit. An enlarged clitoris will likely lead to more sexual pleasure.

As I wrote in Chapter 2, an estrogen supplement in pill form, even when bioidentical, increases your risk of thrombophlebitis, pulmonary embolism, heart attacks, and strokes. Please, do not take oral estrogen. Ever.

How Much Sex is Normal?

Virtually every biological function follows a bell curve, as I previously mentioned. In medicine, we use that curve to define normal. The far ends of the curve—the 2.2 percent of the population at the top and bottom of the curve—are considered abnormally high and low. The 95.6 percent of the population in the middle is defined as normal. How does that relate to your sex drive?

The few people at the bottom of the sex drive spectrum can go for extended periods with no desire for sex of any kind, making them voluntary celibates. The equally small group at the top of the curve are often driven to have sex several times a day, every day of their lives. The majority fall somewhere in between those two extremes.

Sex drive is complicated by the fact that it tends to peak in adolescence when, in our complex culture, early unprotected sex and childbearing can impact our futures in a profoundly negative way. Then, when we are seeking a mate, sex drives go into high gear as we instinctively display our sexual appeal (aka fertility) to potential partners as a means of triggering oxytocin and dopamine bonds. We don't think of it that way, but that's Mother Nature's intent. Within a year or two of obtaining a mate, sexual drive fades to its "normal" baseline.

This can become an issue when romantic partners are mismatched. If one partner is high on the sex drive scale, and the other is significantly lower, the higher drive person will feel deprived and neglected, while the person with the lower drive may feel that unreasonable demands are being made in the bedroom. This is a difficult problem since we're much sexier during the mating game than we will be later in life. People don't lose interest in sex on purpose. It's just part of the way Mother Nature made us.

Restoring Sexual Vitality

Erectile Dysfunction Drugs for Men—and Women Can Use Them Too

There is a class of drugs called phosphodiesterase (PDE) inhibitors. They relax and widen the blood vessels, improving blood flow all over the body, including to the penis, clitoris, and vagina. They're used to treat erectile dysfunction as they make erections easier to achieve and last longer. Clitoral engorgement is also important to female orgasm, as there are five sets of nerves that can trigger an orgasmic response in women. The more of those nerve groups that can be stimulated simultaneously, the more intense the orgasm tends to be. The problem with human anatomy is that it is difficult for one person to trigger more than three of those at one time. But then, that allows for varied techniques and different sets of nerves for different romantic interludes.

PDE inhibitors are also helpful for treating other conditions. They can aid in lowering high blood pressure and treat chronic obstructive pulmonary and heart disease. Increased blood flow in the brain improves cognition and might slow dementia, while increased blood flow to the muscles allows for a better ability to exercise. Since most solid tumors are rich in PDE, a PDE inhibitor will inhibit the growth of breast, colon, and ovarian cancers. (One study showed that the medication Cialis cut the risk of prostate cancer in half).

Three primary drugs target the 11 PDE receptors (PDE5 is the primary receptor that provides erectile function): Viagra, (sildenafil), Levitra, (vardenafil), and Cialis (tadalafil).

- Viagra is the least selective, as it reaches a wide range of PDE receptors. That's also why it has the most side effects, such as red eyes, stuffy nose, and headaches due to increased blood flow to the brain. It takes about 30 minutes to get into your system and lasts only three to four hours.

- Levitra is the most selective for PDE5 with the fewest side effects of the three drugs. It also takes about 30 minutes to activate, but lasts up to 11 hours. Most men take it in the afternoon if they're planning sexual activity in the evening. The problem I have with Viagra and Levitra is that they need to be used when you expect or plan to have sex. One of the joys of a robust sex life is the spontaneous opportunities for intimacy. When my wife calls me at work and asks me to come home at lunch, I know our daughter is in school and it's playtime for the adults.

- Cialis takes about an hour to activate and can last for up to 36 hours. If you take it every day, you won't have to wait 36 hours—you won't have to wait at all. A daily lower dose is the most useful over time. It comes in 2.5-, 5-, 10-, and 20-mg strengths. For those who take it daily, the usual dose starts with 5 mg. After three to five days, the levels of the drug in your bloodstream should be steady, and spontaneous erectile function should be greatly improved.

Cialis is a wonderful daily drug for men who need it. Almost all of our male patients take it because it gives them a better erection even if they don't have erectile dysfunction. It can be just as helpful for many women who take it. It increases vaginal lubrication and offers better clitoral response.

So why don't people know more about these drugs? Because they're approved only for erectile dysfunction in men—doctors and patients don't think they have any off-label benefits.

I don't think a week has gone by when the topic of sexual dysfunction hasn't come up on my radio show. I tell callers that I prefer to prescribe Cialis. It has more side effects, but the 36 hours it lasts and its low daily dose makes it simple, easy, and practical to use. The generic versions are inexpensive, costing only about 50 cents a day.

I've never had any patient respond poorly to these drugs. Some people get mild headaches when they're sexually aroused, but that doesn't stop them from continuing to enjoy sex. Cialis is one of those rare drugs that I'd like to throw in the water supply, so everyone could benefit from it.

The Wonders of Oxytocin

Oxytocin is the happiness and optimism hormone, as mentioned in previous chapters. It makes us look at things positively through what I call rose-tinted oxytocin glasses. It's also one of our bonding hormones, which is why some people refer to it as the "chemical cuddle."

There are several ways to trigger its production:

- Staring into someone's eyes for more than three seconds. That's why lovers gaze at each other's eyes: It triggers oxytocin in both partners.

They don't know that; they only know that it feels good to look at the other person.

- Skin-to-skin contact. Most people love any kind of massage. Someone rubbing your body (whether for muscle relaxation or as part of lovemaking) releases oxytocin and gives you a warm, fuzzy sensation.

- Sexual arousal, especially an orgasm, triggers a huge burst of oxytocin. If sexual frequency decreases, you'll have fewer opportunities to produce oxytocin. Couples who still love each other after many years yet whose sexual contact has diminished will produce less oxytocin because they have less skin-to-skin contact. They spend less time staring into each other's eyes. Eventually the oxytocin just fades away completely, and they become more like roommates than lovers.

When lovers become roommates, oxytocin works to improve moods and intimacy for people of any age. A compounding pharmacist can make oxytocin lozenges that will be slowly dissolved in the cheek, or as a nasal spray. (The nasal spray is more effective, but for people who have chronic colds, allergies, or nasal issues, the lozenges work better.) You stare into someone's eyes, spritz some up your nose, and it works within seconds. Depending on the dose, you can feel good for several hours, and it can be used several times a day. You can also use oxytocin for more than just romantic arousal. It can be extremely helpful for people with previous emotional trauma who have trouble seeing the brighter side of life.

Bear in mind that oxytocin is not an aphrodisiac. It works as an emotional connector that makes you feel better about the person near you and whatever else is going on in your life. It is particularly effective for those with post-traumatic stress syndrome or who've had sexual traumas in their lives. They replay the trauma in their minds so often that it affects both their sexual and platonic relationships. Using oxytocin nasal spray several times a day makes it more difficult to have negative thoughts.

As oxytocin alters your emotions and makes it hard for your brain to go to a negative place, I wish more doctors gave it to their patients, especially as an adjunct to therapy for depression. (The only exception is a contraindication for postpartum depression. For reasons I do not understand, it tends to make postpartum depression worse.) We often prescribe it for couples, especially those who've been together for 35 years or more and whose relationship has become "blah." We ask them how long they've been together; how much romance is in their relationship; and how close they feel to each other. If their answers indicate a need for treatment, oxytocin is often recommended.

Proof Positive of Oxytocin's Usefulness

We had two closely related cases in which oxytocin was the tool that saved a marriage.

A husband in his early 60s and his wife in her late 40s were having difficulty with their relationship. She had been sexually molested in her youth and suffered from PTSD, in which she connected physical intimacy with the assault. Due to their strong religious beliefs, they didn't have sexual relations prior to their marriage After the wedding, when it was time to consummate their sexual relationship, her prior trauma became a stumbling block. In addition to couples counseling, she took oxytocin lozenges twice daily; they help her stop obsessing about her sexual abuse, and she sees her husband's attentions for what they are—an expression of love and caring. Oxytocin did not repair all of her issues, but it helped a lot. As a corollary, we keep her husband's testosterone and DHEA levels a bit lower than usual to avoid driving his libido too high. Her husband loves her as she is, and the most successful strategy, in addition to talk therapy, has been oxytocin.

Another couple who'd been married more than 40 years had no serious issues, but they were slowly drifting apart. They heard me discussing oxytocin on the radio, and decided to see if it might be faster, simpler, and perhaps more effective than couples counseling. It worked! They both use the nasal spray each evening. They make it a point to look into each other's eyes and take two puffs before they cuddle and talk about their day. This isn't a prelude to passion since that aspect of their lives faded some time ago.

They report that the "oxy ritual," as they call it, has made their lives much better, and that they feel closer to one another than they have for years.

Oxytocin for Non-Orgasmic Women

Oxytocin is also a medication used to help pregnant women when labor is not progressing as it should. In those situations, oxytocin is given intravenously, and the uterus begins to contract, which speeds up the delivery process. The idea struck me a few years ago: Why don't we put oxytocin in a vaginal gel, inject it into the vagina to the cervix so that it can be absorbed into the uterus, thereby making the uterus hypersensitive during sex and more likely to trigger orgasmic spasms? This method works for about 30 percent of the women who use it. For women who are already orgasmic, they can become multi-orgasmic. The medication also acts as a lubricant. The gel that our pharmacist concocts is sweet, so it tastes good during oral sex. If your gynecologist works with a compounding pharmacy, you might want to give this a try. It can be a lifesaver when having sex.

Normally, oxytocin does not cross intact skin. But many men find that when their partner has oxytocin gel in her vagina, his sensitivity, hence his orgasmic response, is enhanced. My best guess is that this is since the skin on the penis is quite thin, and the warmth and friction of sexual activity coupled with the vagina filled with oxytocin may indeed drive enough of the drug into his system to cause this effect. Another explanation is that her improved responsiveness might be enough of a turn-on to enhance his experience.

Dopamine, Serotonin, and Your Libido

The neurotransmitter dopamine is our addiction and pleasure hormone. Positron emission scans have demonstrated that the same areas of the brain light up when people are shown photographs of the partner they love as they do for cocaine and heroin addiction. They are literally addicted to that human being, which helps explain why some people have severe reactions to a breakup. They're suddenly in a withdrawal-like state from an addiction to the other person. It's not that they want to act out in any way, but at least there's a biological reason.

In a romantic relationship, the oxytocin and dopamine tend to work in tandem to enhance the relationship and keep partners interested in each other. Over time, sexual frequency tends to decline, so oxytocin levels fall, but the elevated dopamine levels and desire to stay together may increase over time.

That said, for most people, dopamine receptors decline as you age. This explains why people get less pleasure out of life in general, affecting their libido along with everything else. There are dopamine agonist medications that increase levels, but they can trigger destructive addictive behaviors. People can become gambling addicts or sexually promiscuous because they're looking for their next dopamine hit.

Serotonin, the happiness and optimism neurotransmitter hormone, is a mixed blessing. High levels give us a sense of well-being. Very low levels impart depression, fatigue, and lethargy. Amphetamines (drugs that speed up your mind and body and keep you awake) and medications that dramatically raise serotonin levels make you feel wonderful. You can accomplish anything. You can't fail. The world is great, until you realize you're addicted and need more and more of the drugs lest you come down hard off the serotonin high and things start to fall apart.

Amphetamine addicts often become addicted to sex, and many of them lose weight. Prozac and most of the serotonin uptake inhibitors often improve mood, but cause weight gain and suppress libido. Wellbutrin, on the other hand, has been documented to increase the incidence of women becoming more sexually active and enjoying multiple orgasms. All things being equal, I would rather a psychiatrist prescribe Wellbutrin than Prozac.

We do not prescribe any of these medications in our clinics due to how easily they can trigger addictive behaviors, cause weight gain, and require a long, often difficult, tapering-off period for those who want or need to stop taking them.

How Dopamine Genetics Affect Sexual Behavior

Not far from Denver, Colorado, live two populations of burrowing ground rodents, the prairie voles. They are physiologically indistinguishable, at least on the gross level. They look and act the same. Their diet, nesting structures, and environment are essentially identical. But one population mates for life and, in fact, the voles do so after only a single act of copulation. The other population is wildly polyamorous.

Scientists studying these prairie voles found a difference in the dopamine receptors in their brains. (A quick genetics lesson: We have genes that code for both hormones and hormone receptors in our bodies. Mammals, including us, have five different dopamine receptors and five different genes that code for the production of those receptors. We designate them DR for Dopamine Receptor, and number them D1-D5. When you see DRD1, it means Dopamine Receptor D1. Our DNA usually has several repetitions of important genes in case something happens to damage a portion of the DNA where that gene is coded. But the number of repeated gene coding varies from individual to individual.) DRD2 seems to be the trigger for that initial and long-term bonding between a couple. Once that bonding takes place, if you have a load of DRD1 receptors active, it makes you reject approaches from other sexual partners.

The DRD4 tells a very different tale. Animals, including humans, with few DRD4 repeats in their genome are monogamous, or nearly so. Those with more DRD4 repeats search out more partners, even if they are already mated.

The scientists started looking at other animals who mate for life, like swans, and found that those with long-term mating behavior have very few DRD4 repeats in their genome, and those with lots of repeats do not mate for life. Often, they take a mate, but also have sex with others in addition to their chosen partner. Then the scientists looked at humans. We have at least 23 different variants of DRD4 genome repeats. It wasn't surprising to see that people with high numbers of repeats have high divorce rates because they are more likely to be physically incapable of remaining monogamous. They emotionally might *want* to be faithful, and they often struggle with this, but they're the ones who cheat and say, "I don't know why I did it"—because they don't. (Not a suitable excuse, of course.) People with very few repeats tend to be those couples who meet in high school, have been together forever, are never tempted to stray, and live happy lives together. Most of us are somewhere in between those variations in DRD4 repeats.

Those with more than seven repeats often display impulsive behaviors. In addition to sexual adventures, they tend to take financial, social, and romantic risks and engage in risky sports. DRD3 and DRD5 are both involved in emotional attachments and movement/coordination. Mutations in these receptors tend to induce schizophrenia.

What we usually think of as our ability to make choices can be strongly influenced by our genetic makeup.

Being Open About Your Sexual Needs as You Get Older

There is still much shame and embarrassment about being honest and open about sexual needs. So many of my patients have a hard time talking about it. I have equal numbers of female and male physicians on staff, so patients can talk more easily with a same-gender practitioner, if they prefer. My hope is that people will come to understand that sexuality, like eating, is a natural function. It feels good to eat when you're hungry and it should feel good to have sex.

When I'm doing my radio show and the inevitable questions about sexual performance and sexuality come up, I explain that there is a big difference between romance and erotic desire. I say that romance is the deep emotional connection with another human being along with the desire to please and give each other pleasure. The erotic desire is physical passion. It's wonderful if you can have both in your life, but if nature, time, and disease eliminated most of the erotic, the romantic is still there and it's the romance that will keep you in love.

I also discuss how overusing the internet and/or interacting on social media has distorted a lot of things, such as body image. Filters make it ridiculously easy to alter your face and body, so people can look the way you want to look, rather than how they actually look. The internet also makes it easier to shop for things you once had to buy only in stores. When I was a teenager, overloaded with testosterone, pharmacies wouldn't sell condoms if you weren't at least 21. That led to some creative strategizing! Fortunately, those days are long-gone. Now you can buy sex toys or other paraphernalia in the privacy of your home. Doctors at our clinics encourage our patients to explore their sexuality when their libidos make a welcome return.

She Knew What She Wanted

When I asked a new patient, a 32-year-old woman, why she was seeing us at her young age, her response set me back a bit. She said, "My husband's a trust fund manager and I'm his second trophy wife. I want to make damn sure I am his last. So, keep me as hot as you can, as long as you can." I explained that our clinic didn't offer plastic surgery services. We addressed the normal but undesired changes of aging. Once I was sure that she understood what we do, I put her on the same program as my wife. This patient was already fit and lean and went to great lengths to care for her body on the assumption that doing so would maintain her husband's interest.

Now, more than 20 years later, she's in her mid-50s and still married to the same guy. Either our efforts have paid off as she expected, or they grew up a lot as a couple. Let's hope it was some of each.

The social media distortions leading to the body dysmorphia that plague many younger people are less of an issue for our patients. They recognize that their bodies are not what they once were and most of them have come to grips with that. They're less likely to make comparisons to younger people. If they're still feeling bad about how they look, I share a story. Many years ago, I was driving with a girlfriend north of Santa Monica. At the top of a hill, we looked down and saw a small group of people frolicking and playing volleyball on a lovely stretch of beach. We decided to join them, so we made our way down, and as we arrived, I stopped dead. Before us were some of the most beautiful naked people I had ever seen. I don't know if they were with a modeling agency, or what, but all the women were breathtakingly gorgeous, and all the men were spectacularly buff. I suddenly felt old and fat and ugly. I know I've said not to make comparisons, but in this case, it was impossible not to. We turned around and slowly walked back up the hill in silence.

Sometimes, that's not convincing enough, because I understand that how you feel about your body can make you inhibited about having sex, especially with a new partner. I have deep scars on both arms and legs and my chest. I've said for decades that 99 percent of humans look better with their clothes on than off, and the other 1 percent never made it to my office. I can say that with a laugh because I'm part of the 99 percent!

Banding and I were in love before we spent our first night together, yet I was extremely nervous about getting undressed. I'd previously told her about my many scars, puckers, and lines that aren't supposed to be there, but there's a difference between telling and seeing. As we prepared to spend our first night together, I reminded her of my scarred body and told her that I hoped it would not bother her too much. She said, "Let me decide what I think." She unbuttoned and took off my shirt, then undid my belt and dropped my trousers around my ankles. She walked around my body, running her fingers over some of the bigger and uglier puckers and scars. Then, returning to my front, she looked up into my eyes and said, "Those are a warrior's scars. They make me feel safe because I know you'll fight to protect what you love."

An Oscar-winning Hollywood screenwriter could not have scripted that better. I wanted to marry her on the spot. Believe me when I say how lucky and thankful I am that she said that, because it was the last time I ever worried about how my scars and old wounds look. Knowing that she accepts me as I am, not as I wish I were, is powerful validation of me as a flawed human being, but one still worthy of loving and being loved by a wonderful woman.

What we do discuss with people who come to the clinic is *not* about how fat makes people look (which can be perceived as fat-shaming) but the all-important need to get rid of the fat that's interfering with the rest of their body's functions and harming their health.

Once the weight comes off, the systemic inflammation declines, and hormone levels improve, many patients wake up sexually again. Some say, "You know, I look pretty good compared to where I was." Even if the changes are minimal, simply believing they look better makes them *feel* better, and when they feel better, that often makes them more willing to be adventurous with their partner. But the partners need to be willing and able, or there will be trouble in paradise.

You already learned that sexual desire is a continuum. Some folks like, or even need, a lot of sex; others not so much. We had a couple of relatively young folks at our clinic who exemplified the trouble this mismatch can cause. Kate was on her second marriage. The first fell apart because her ex-husband ran off with another woman. When she met her current husband, she was impressed by his deep religious nature and his respect for her, manifested by the fact that he never tried to have sex with her before they were married. For me, that last bit was a red flag. Remember what I said about people becoming sexually hyperactive during the mating/dating period? Well, it turned out that he did not want sex after the marriage either. Kate had a healthy libido, and during her previous marriage had been used to sex about twice a week, which is about par for healthy, mid-range-sex-drive people. Her new husband worked hard, provided for her and her children from her previous marriage, and was kind and respectful, but sex was simply not something he thought about or especially desired. They would have sex once a month at the most, and at other times once every two or three months. Kate loved him. She had no desire to leave him, but she was not sure she could live the rest of her life in an essentially sexless relationship.

We checked him out. He was totally healthy. Fine hormone levels and no pathology we could find anywhere. He was simply a low-drive person when it came to sex. His desire for marriage was based on companionship and being able to share his thoughts, dreams, and feelings with another person. Even during his youth, he had a very low sex drive.

Kate did not want to have sex with anyone else, and she opted to stay in the marriage and to focus her energies on her career while trying her best to ignore her erotic urges. Did she make the "right" choice? Will she be able to happily live a sexless life? I have my doubts. But then, it is not my choice or judgment to make.

A man or woman unable or unwilling to have sex during that initial mating period is sending a strong message about their erotic drive, or rather the lack of it. Kate should have paid attention, but the reality is that she, like most adult Americans, had never been educated about human sexuality. We teach our kids about the mechanics of sex. We may teach them the moral beliefs of our personal religious traditions. We may well even teach them about pregnancy, sexually transmitted diseases, and contraception. But the actual realities of human biology/psychology and relationships are totally ignored.

When Libido Goes a Little . . . Well, You Decide!

Because what we do for people often enhances their desire and capacity for romance and sex, the clinic came to the attention of a local private swingers' club. Folks go there to have sex with their mates and/or strangers of their choosing. At first, I was surprised when I learned that our clinic had become well-known among the club-goers. When I thought about it, the connection was obvious. My professional morality is simple: If it hurts my patient, it is bad. If it helps my patient, it is good. Other than that, I go to great lengths not to judge other people's lives. But the notion of 200 assorted people having sex with many strangers strikes me as the way to catch several sexually transmitted diseases in one evening!

In another situation, a 63-year-old businesswoman called on a Monday, distressed that her hormone balance had gotten out of line, and she was having menstrual-like bleeding. This happens occasionally, and our doctors are good at fixing this by adjusting hormone levels. What caused us to raise our eyebrows was when she told us that her bleeding had to be stopped by Friday because her "club" had a charter flight to an island resort. Half of the flight was going to be men, and she planned to have sex with as many of them as possible during the ten-day trip.

In this case it was very difficult not to judge!

When a Reawakened Libido Can Be a Problem

I've had to inform some of our younger female doctors new to our clinics that they'll be treating many men, especially older ones, who've had no sex drive for decades. When their libidos wake up, these guys often don't know how to handle it and act inappropriately. It's as if they're adolescents again, and can go from being silly to being offensive with sexual innuendos and sexual aggressions. Such behavior with staff members is unacceptable. All these patients are reminded of the things they learned the first time around when they were teenagers. But in some rare, extreme situations, they find themselves no longer welcome at the clinic. My physicians understand the situation and know how to gently, but clearly, set appropriate boundaries.

We much prefer to work with and enjoy patients like Elise, an 81-year-old who went on a vacation to the Caribbean. When she returned and I checked her blood work, her hormone levels were way off. "What happened?" I asked her. "Your values were great when you left."

"Well, doc," she said with a saucy smile. "I gotta admit I had to drop off the DHEA and testosterone because the damn pool boy was so hot, I was sure I was going to get myself in trouble."

I'd like every woman to feel this good, but that's not always possible, especially if chronic illnesses interfere with sexual functioning. This can be a problem for couples if one person's libido returns and the other's doesn't. The dichotomy is often that men are still interested in sex, but they can't perform. Women can perform, but they've lost interest—unless they choose to start treatment to improve their libido.

Many of our patients come to us depressed about their sex life or lack thereof. Those whose health is not optimal tend to have hormonally triggered depression and anxiety. If they had active, productive, and optimistic lives until perimenopause, when their hormone levels dropped, that can almost always be fixed. But if they're still depressed once their testosterone and other hormones are increased, and they're losing weight and physically active, counseling is recommended. There's no age limit for seeing a therapist and getting the help you deserve.

Recommended Supplements for Libido

Refer to Chapter 5 for more details. Discuss the proper doses for your needs as well any potential contraindications with your doctor before taking any new supplements.

Astaxanthin This carotenoid improves all muscle function. It is the reddish-orange pigment in salmon, giving them almost supernatural strength and endurance on their upstream journey to spawn. Clinical studies show that taking 10 mg or more a day can increase strength significantly in older people.

Quercetin In addition to being a great antioxidant, this polyphenol inhibits the formation of senescent cells, increases cellular energy, and suppresses allergic reactions.

Resveratrol This anti-inflammatory antioxidant decreases your risk of dying from a heart attack and also improves the quality of your skin and decreases the formation of senescent cells.

Vitamins C, E, and K Potent anti-inflammatories that decrease senescent cell formation, these vitamins are good antioxidants that decrease cancer cell formation, help the immune systems fight infections, and give us stronger, more flexible bones.

Part III

How to Live

Chapter 11

Stress Management

We all have to deal with stress; it's part of life. Nobody goes through life without encountering some problems. Do you worry about your future? Do you have concerns about money? How is your family doing? Do you have sleepless nights, tossing and turning because you can't stop thinking about problems at home or work? Are you afraid of dying? Do you read the obituaries every day and think you're next?

I tell my patients that the "good old days" were really the bad old days. Life was difficult and dangerous. There were no antibiotics or antivirals, so infection usually meant death. Smoke from fires damaged lungs. Women and their babies frequently died in childbirth; with a 50/50 chance a child who survived birth would die before age five. Since birth control didn't exist for the average woman, sex usually resulted in pregnancy; on average, every sixth or seventh pregnancy was fatal. Our stressors seem big to us, but those who lived in the bad old days would have loved to have had our first-world problems.

I see so many patients who are burdened by the weight of the modern world. So many of them tell me they don't know how to cope anymore. I tell them about the effect of stress hormones (see Chapter 2) and that there are simple strategies to implement in their daily lives that will help. They deserve to feel their best. I've talked to countless seniors who are constantly doing things for others while neglecting themselves. When I ask why, they say don't feel they're worth it. They refuse to ask for help because they "don't want to be a bother." I hasten to add that being able to say "No!" is a yes from me!

For all her cunning, Mother Nature did program us humans to be able to withstand a lot of acute, or short-term, emotional and physical stress. But many of the stresses we have in our modern world are of our own creation. Anxiety, fear, and feelings of failure are created by our brains when we don't get enough of the supporting hormones we need and our bodies have too much fat we don't need. We need to kick you back to your enthusiastic, adolescent self who wants to climb that mountain again.

Changing how you think about yourself and what you deserve is an enormous step toward minimizing your stress. Adding self-care—mindfulness techniques and taking care of your skin and body—to your daily to-do list is equally important.

Stress Management Is an All-Day Mindset—So Look at It as an Opportunity

When I was a soldier, we were taught to manage stress by being aggressive on the battlefield. My natural optimism kicked in when we were in combat and things were going wrong. Instead of worrying if I was going to die, I recognized ways to get around the enemy fire so I could do my job. Thank God those years are behind me, but I've come to realize that I still behave the same way when I'm stressed. I don't freeze. I don't get angry. I don't get anxious. My mantra is: I'm being sent a new opportunity. Figure out what to do with it.

I don't expect you to say, "I'm being sent a new opportunity" when your car is rear-ended or someone you love becomes ill. What I hope you will consider is that trying to have a more optimistic mindset—the kind that will last all day, or better yet, all day, every day—can help to minimize your reactions to stressful situations. It's only human nature to lurch into catastrophizing from time to time, thinking, *If this happens, then that will happen and then the next thing and they're all bad*, and before you know it, it's World War III and we're all going to die because they brought the wrong creamer for your coffee.

I spent several decades struggling, exhausted, and stressed when I was a country doctor. But even then, I was always looking for innovative and sometimes off-the-wall ways to make my patients' lives better. That's *why* I do what I do—my approach to longevity is to make every patient's life as good as it can possibly be. If I am exercising, my goal is to get as strong and fast and limber as I can. What if I become injured? My goal becomes, *How do I heal this as quickly and as completely as possible?* I don't accept negative outcomes. So how can you manage your stress about your longevity and not have your stress manage you?

The number one thing to know is that there's nothing wrong with you. What you're living with right now is not what you have to live with. Perhaps you have a dim view of life. You have a short temper. You are tired all the time. You are grumpy. Guess what? *You are normal.* You are exactly how Mother Nature made you to be at this stage of your life.

If you don't like what you see in the mirror, or don't care to continue being the current version of you, then take the steps outlined in this book to become who you do want to be. When you raise your hormone levels, when you lose the fat, when you move your body regularly—you will find you are no longer fearful and glum. You will be more optimistic and will feel energized to do the things you now know will make your life better. You do have the ability to make these changes and stick to them.

People call into my radio show and say, "Dr. Mixon, I want to be you. You're always so cheerful and optimistic." I'm happy to be that way. I try to get as much joy as I can out of life for as long as I can. This is what I tell my callers: "Yes, you are going to die. But guess what? So am I. I might get hit by a bus this afternoon. We're all going to die. But guess what? I've got a whole lot of stuff I want to do first. And when I die, I suspect I'm going to be disappointed that I left half a dozen jobs undone."

Stress = opportunities. I see this response every day at work thanks to my company president, Lynn Kasel. When a problem or a crisis arise and most businesspeople (even me!) might respond by saying, "How am I going to fix it? What's it going to cost? Whom do I have to hire? How long before it gets resolved?" Lynn, on the other hand, finds a way to see the positive in every crisis and make every stumble profitable. He is invariably optimistic. He looks at the problem and his default response is not "How am I going to fix this?" but "It's not a problem. It's a challenge. It's an opportunity. Well, we didn't plan on that happening, but we can turn that into something else." And he does!

I have trouble thinking like Lynn at work, but nowhere else. I almost never think of other situations as problems. I observe them and ask what I can learn from them and how can I make things better as a result.

That's why Rule #6 is "If you try you might fail, but if you refuse to try, you're a failure." If you try, you might not succeed, but you will learn from your experience. That's not failure. But if you don't try, you'll never know what might have happened. Thomas Edison said, "I didn't fail 1,000 times. The light bulb was an invention with 1,000 steps." Or maybe he meant the battery. Sources vary about the exact quote, but the point remains the same: If he did fail 999 times, he didn't see it that way because on the thousandth try, he was no longer a failure. And he changed the world.

Dealing with Your Mental Health as You Get Older

Our emotions are just as real as our physical bodies. You can't see or touch them, but, by God, you can feel them. Acknowledging them isn't easy. I've lost count of how many patients have said "I'm fine" when it was obvious they were struggling. It's not surprising that mental health issues like depression and anxiety are more common in older people.

There are two reasons for this. The first is that as many people get older, their health issues increase—hopefully, yours will decrease after reading and using this book!—and their energy levels plummet. We live in an ageist society where we're judged by our wrinkles, hair loss, and bulging bellies, and found wanting. Or we're not seen at all. We become invisible to those who see youth as the marker for success rather than venerating the wisdom and experience of their elders. For those who were successful in their professional fields, no longer being regarded as a player can be devastating. Loved ones and colleagues are getting sick and dying. Grief and heartbreak take an enormous toll on the psyche. Of course, people are going to be sad, depressed, and anxious as a result.

The second reason is something I explained in previous chapters. Some mental health issues arise due to our hormones. The so-called sex hormones are closely related to our sexuality in our late adolescence as we develop our reproductive capacity. But once the job of procreation is done, the primary function of those hormones is to act as neurotransmitters. Our brains' hormones affect how we see ourselves and the world around us. They are a part of what gives us our stress tolerance, confidence, ability to put up with opposition, enthusiasm, and ability to laugh at the absurdities of life.

One of the reasons we get grumpy, short-tempered, and set in our ways as we get older is the declining production of hormones in our bodies and the resulting shortage of those hormones in our brains. A man who was used to coping with stress will find that such challenges become harder to handle as he gets older. Without the proper hormonal balance, he will have two responses: He will withdraw from life, or he will lash out in anger because he's scared. He'll become intolerant of change or of anything that makes him uncomfortable. What a waste of his remaining years!

If your mental state is becoming increasingly upsetting, working with an experienced and understanding therapist is an excellent idea, but that alone is not what you need. If you have an acute condition, bear in mind that only some medical professionals, such as psychiatrists and NDs, can prescribe drugs that might help. Use as many of the self-care strategies you'll read about in this chapter as you can. But you know by now that putting the hormones of your youth back in your brain is as crucial a step as advice and/or meds from a competent mental health practitioner.

Many of our patients have been successful in businesses of one sort or another. Some of them are retired, while others are still fully employed. A recurring theme among our small business owners and executives is that they felt unable to cope and needed to retire. Or equally bad, they felt pushed out because the ageist people around them no longer believed they were up to the job. I have had several small business folks who, once we restored their hormones, discovered that they were not ready to quit and ended up going out and starting a new business while others their age were sitting around reminiscing about their past glories.

In his early 60s, a patient named Alfred was bought out of his small business. He was tired of the constant stress and frustrations of owning and running the place anyway. He thought he would spend his remaining days playing golf and visiting his grandkids. But his kids and grandchildren had their own busy lives, and after a few years as a patient with us and much-improved health, his drive to achieve returned, and he was tired of feeling like a has-been. Ten years after his buy-out he went back to work full time and ended up buying out the folks who bought him out.

I understand his desire to keep working. I opened the first Longevity Medical Clinic at 50. Then I started what is now the Relief Factor company at 65. I opened a medical spa at 70. At 76, I've written this book and I'm looking at taking some of my enterprises national. Retire? Never even considered it. I'm having way too much fun!

You can see my gray hair and wrinkles—I earned them!—but my brain is still functioning with the neurotransmitters of a young man. Because I have the hormonal balance of a 25-year-old, I also have the self-confidence, drive, energy, and ambition of a 25-year-old, coupled with the life experience of a 76-year-old. Come on, world, I'm ready for you!

Resilience: Your New Favorite Word

I define resilience as the ability to adjust to new and unexpected circumstances. Most of the time we connect that with something negative: Something bad happens and we need to to deal with what has been thrown at us. But it has a flip side that is often ignored. Opportunities also arise that are totally unexpected, and resilience comes into play there too. It is what allows us to readjust our expectations and plans to take advantage of the changes and prosper.

What I have learned is that opportunities often come disguised as a problem. With the proper mix of hormones in our brains, we are better prepared to look through the problem and find the opportunity hiding below. There is a degree of inborn capacity for responding to stress. But losing the hormonal support in your brain takes whatever your inborn level was and crashes it to the ground.

"My mother is such a worry wart about everything," my patient Jonathan told me. "Her cousin Will's daughter Janelle invited us to lunch a few weeks after Will died. When we got to Janelle's house, she wasn't there. I was pissed. My mother sat down on the stoop and said, 'I bet she's dead.' I said, 'Mom, she's not dead. I bet she just forgot.'" About 20 minutes later, Janelle drives up and sees us. Her face was a picture. Of course, she forgot about inviting us to lunch. My mother has spent her entire life leaping to the worst possible scenarios. When my kids go see their friends, she freaks out if I don't know where they are every minute. I remind her that when I was little, there were no cellphones, and I'd go out to play, and parents trusted us to be smart enough to take care of ourselves."

I wish I could sit down with Jonathan's mother and talk with her about resilience. I'd explain to her that when she is in a stressful situation and those fight-or-flight hormones kick in, being better aware of her default responses (anxiety and catastrophizing) would help her be able to minimize them.

While having a conversation about decision making with a colleague who is a neuro-psychiatrist, he told me, "Jerry, some of us are just not wired to cope with stress. No matter what happens to *you*, you're resilient, where other people just crumble. In my practice, I deal with those who crumble. There's no way to explain it. And there's no way to know why some do and some don't."

I respect my neuro-psychiatrist friend, but I remember being emotionally and physically at the end of my rope when I was a burnt-out country doctor. Whatever emotional strength and resilience I had in my youth had faded by the age of 50. But after restoring my hormone levels to a youthful range, they returned in full force.

We all know people who are oiled like ducks—problems just seem to roll off them. I saw that in combat situations. When we shipped off to Vietnam, everybody in our unit wanted to be there. We had been well-trained and were ready for combat, yet when the shooting started, some of my buddies could not lift their faces out of the mud. They *wanted* to be brave. They *wanted* to be soldiers. They were incapable of doing what they thought they'd be able to do. They weren't cowards; they just didn't have that inborn ability to respond to the stressful situation of having enemy soldiers trying to kill them.

Every animal has some version of the flight-or-fight response. If you startle a rabbit, it will freeze for a second or two, then take off. Most humans are the same way; when danger suddenly strikes, we freeze for a moment. The bravest and best combat soldier I ever met was Charlie Morris. He never froze even for an instant. The second the shooting started; he was headed for the guns. When I asked him if he was afraid, he told me that, of course, he was always scared, but he refused to let fear keep him from doing his job. Unlike Charlie, with that first crack of a rifle or first explosive impact, I froze for what sometimes seemed like hours. I knew objectively that it was no more than a fraction of a second, and then I got moving and did my job. Some guys froze for two or three seconds, then broke loose. Some guys just froze. They literally could not get up and move toward the danger.

No matter how much you want to be a warrior, whether in war or in peace, if you're not, you're not. That's okay. One of life's most important lessons is to learn who you are. Who is that person in the mirror? Recognizing and acknowledging who you are physically, emotionally, and intellectually is an automatic stress-buster. Once you do, you can set about making changes. You can make good decisions when you are dealing with the world as it really is rather than some fantasy version of reality.

That notion is critical. The world is what it is and it is seldom what we would like it to be, or what philosophers or politicians tell us it should be. It just is. If we want to be successful in any aspect of our lives, we need to recognize and learn to deal with reality. That is first and foremost the reality of who we are! Then, look at the external realities that we face. The next step is to realistically assess our resources, both our own and those of the people we can recruit to help us. Only then can we get to work and do the work.

Accept your limitations and embrace them. We need poets, artists, warriors, and managers. We also need people to do the things that need doing, like the staff at my supplement fulfillment center who send out thousands of packages every day.

Be the most joyful, happiest, most fulfilled person that you can be.

The Stress of Dealing with Death

On the Holmes and Rahe stress scale from 1 to 100, created by two psychiatrists, the Impact Score of the death of a spouse is 100. Divorce is 73; Christmas approaching is 12, which shows that any event in life can be stressful!

As you get older, the loss of your loved ones, colleagues, and friends can be especially difficult to process when somebody who you thought was healthy dies suddenly. You think, "Am I next?" You can become fearful and depressed. Memories from when you and the deceased were young, vital, and full of hopes and plans for the future can trigger emotions that range from momentary sadness to long periods of depression. Ongoing and relentless mourning creates stress that can make an enormous, negative impact on your immune system and wear you down.

There are powerful connections between our emotional centers and our immune response. People do die of a broken heart! Some parents never fully recover from the loss or serious injury to a child. And the death of a long-term mate can destroy the rest of the survivor's life, profoundly affecting both their physical and emotional health. People with whom you have a strong and/or a long-term bond impact your life for both good and ill.

Joy and gratitude are powerful boosters of both mood and physical resilience. Sorrow and depression do the opposite. Developing a habit of looking for the good and the positive in every situation can have a potent impact on your long-term health.

The men from my 173rd Airborne team are almost all gone now. Reunions for surviving soldiers are occasionally held, but I've never attended one. I don't want to see what life has done to the brave young men I served with, who were once so fantastically fit and full of life. And I owe my life and the joys I have been granted for the past 50 years to their dedication to duty. But I know that the character traits that made us good soldiers didn't necessarily translate into success in civilian life. I've been afraid to see what happened to them. That has been one of my few real fears. I just can't bear to see them.

How Heartbreak Can Age You

Grief isn't just an internal emotion; it can be palpably visible on the faces of the bereaved and in their movements. I've had the sad task of talking to families who've just lost a loved one. They literally can visibly age overnight. As time goes by, I hope they will recover some of their vibrancy, but many don't.

Many people don't realize that grief seems contagious. It hits your doctors, too. Physicians and other medical workers are taught to keep emotional distances from patients to protect ourselves from burning out when dealing with people who are sick, frightened, or in pain. The job can kill you, as evidenced by the fact that the suicide rate for doctors is far higher than for the general population. As a country doctor, I had to tell parents that their child had died, or that their beloved spouse had a terminal disease, or that they themselves were suffering from an incurable condition that would limit or end their lives. I have wrapped a sobbing patient in my arms and wept with them more than once, my heart breaking for their pain and fear and for my inability to help them. Such a situation is designed to force a physician to confront the limits of human knowledge. We doctors hate not knowing. We hate not being able to help! We go into medicine because we have a deep-seated need to nurture, protect, and help those in need. But life and death have a way of reminding us that MD does not stand for minor deity.

There is a temporary heart condition known as Takotsubo cardiomyopathy, or broken-heart syndrome, first described in 1990 in Japan. More than 90 percent of the reported cases are found in women. Some sufferers were thought to have had heart attacks when it was this disorder instead. Most recover fully, but some cardiac symptoms can persist, and a few die of a quite literally broken heart. Grief should never be downplayed or dismissed as something to "get over."

People often think of the body and the brain as two separate entities, along with our emotional state as a third intangibility. But the brain is a part of the body, not a separate entity, and our emotions are generated by the brain, and are a critical signal about its health. Truly healthy people are more likely happy people. Healthy people are usually sexual creatures who enjoy the sensuality of romance, love, and passion. I say usually, because, as pointed out in Chapter 10, there is a wide range of "normal" when it comes to erotic feelings.

I'm not afraid of dying. I'm familiar with death—violent deaths from my youth and the natural deaths of my patients from more than 50 years practicing medicine. As a physician, I have been with many people as they left this world. I was sometimes the only person available to sit and hold someone's hand or stroke their cheek and let them know that someone cared as they lay dying.

One patient was a lovely gentleman in his early 80s, a widower who remarried after his wife died decades earlier. He had half a dozen diseases, any of which could have killed him. He was in the hospital yet again, but he didn't seem any sicker to me than he had been on previous hospitalizations. When a nurse called me and asked, "This patient says he's going to die at two o'clock this afternoon, and he wants me to bring his family in. What should I do?" I told her to call the family. It would be a nice visit if he doesn't die, and if he does, he may know something you and I don't. His family all came, and he gave some last bequests. Then he turned to his current wife and said, "Honey, I want you to know that my first wife is standing right over here, and she wants me to tell you how grateful she is for the care and love you've given me in the years since she's been gone. When it's your turn to come, the two of us will be there to welcome you." Then he turned on his side and died.

Hospice workers often have similar experiences with the dying, who carry on conversations or have visitations with people only they can see. I'm mentioning this as it has convinced me that when we leave this earth, we continue in some form. It's comforting and stress-relieving. I don't want to leave Banding, Ivory, my older children, and my work because I'm having a wonderful time. I'd like to stick around as long as I practically can, but if I become a burden and incapable of caring for those I love,

I would like to go. I'm certain that I will still look over them from the other side, wherever that happens to be.

Self-Care Strategies to Minimize Stress

Maximize Mindfulness

I suggest to my patients that they find some sort of mindfulness technique and use it daily. Whether it's controlled breathing, meditation, or journaling, it's a matter of finding the one that resonates with you so you will want to use it all the time. The more you practice mindfulness, the easier it will be for you to calm yourself and move on when you find yourself in stressful situations.

Here are some mindfulness ideas that have been helpful to many of my patients:

Controlled breathing: This sounds simple, but it does work. Sit in a quiet place without distractions. Breathe in for a count of three, then breathe out for a count of four (or any combination you like). Repeat several times, until you feel better. This will slow down your pulse rate. If you take yoga or Pilates classes, you will be taught about controlled breathing that will aid in relaxation.

I taught this technique to my daughter Ivory during the morning piano lesson I give her. When she had difficulty with a particular passage, she'd become agitated and start pounding and banging the keys. I taught her to stop, put her hands in her lap, and take a slow, deep breath in for three counts, then out for four counts, and repeat until she calmed down. I explained that no one can do a complex task when they are angry, frustrated, or discouraged. Being calm and relaxed allows focus, and focus allows you to achieve.

Systemic muscular relaxation: Gently move your head from side to side. Then moving down, identify each part of your body. While concentrating on that specific part, say aloud: *My neck is relaxing . . . my shoulders are relaxing . . . my arms are relaxing . . . my fingers are relaxing.* Do this down your entire body until you feel calmer and looser.

Stand up and stretch: You already know how good this can make you feel. Go back to page 168 in Chapter 7 for tips.

Meditation: Clearing your mind with focused concentration is an automatic stress-buster. Many forms of meditation have been used for thousands of years, including prayer, which is one of the most powerful forms of meditation I know. You can meditate almost anywhere for any amount of time. You can do it at your desk at work when you have a quiet moment, in a comfortable spot in your home, or even try a moving meditation by going for a walk. (Walking meditations are best done silently or by listening to music without lyrics, which can be distracting.) Guided meditations are helpful for many, as they often combine meditation with controlled breathing. You can find guided meditations on YouTube, and there are many apps as well.

A daily mantra: Not a day goes by that I don't express my gratitude to my creator. I simple say, "Thank you, God" many times. I say it when appreciating the beauty of the rabbits and birds I encounter during my morning jogs on the Kirkland Trail. I say it when seeing people less vigorous than myself as well as when the speedy college athletes from Northwest University run past me up the hill. Does that make it a mantra or a prayer? I'm not sure. Some of each, I guess. I just know that I am grateful for my wonderful life, and it only seems fitting to tell God "thank you."

Your mantra can be anything that resonates with you. (If you have taken a Transcendental Meditation course, you were given a mantra that is sacred and unique to you.) Many of my patients have told me that they came up with a personal mantra when they were having a difficult time. "When I was having radiation after my surgery for breast cancer, my mantra was 'It could be worse,'" my patient Julianna told me. "I was lucky that my cancer was caught early. While sitting in the radiation waiting room at the hospital, I saw other patients, all of whom seemed to be in far worse shape than I was, and I would repeat my mantra to minimize my stress. To this day, when something stupid or stressful happens, I tell myself, *It could be worse*, because that is invariably true."

Keep a journal: While computers are marvels, nothing beats a handwritten diary or journal that encourages you to slow down and express your thoughts and feelings on paper.

Aromatherapy: Smelling anything goes through your olfactory nerves directly to your brain. Perfume, candles, flowers, or essential oils with your favorite herb or flower will instantly make you feel better. Using a diffuser with aromatherapy oils will scent your environment. You can choose oils that have uplifting, energizing, or calming effects. Wild lavender grows along the sidewalks and trails in our area. I often pinch off a bloom or two and squish them between my fingers to enjoy the delightful scent the lavender oil leaves on my skin.

Rituals: Doing the same things that you know makes you feel good is one of the great pleasures in life. Banding and I have an evening ritual that soothes us both. While Ivory is having her evening piano lesson, Banding and I take a walk together. Rain, shine, snow—it doesn't matter. We bundle up and walk side by side for an hour or so and hold hands. We share our thoughts and feelings about whatever happened that day. When we return home, we spend an hour with Ivory before she goes to bed. Then Banding and I snuggle down and get ready for sleep. Since we are usually up and going by 5 a.m., bedtime for us is between 9 to 10 p.m.

Take Care of Your Skin

Mother Nature made sure that anyone who passes their sell-by date is going to show it. Skin sags, lines appear, wrinkles deepen, brown spots pop up, and hair falls out. Looking in the mirror and seeing an aging face when you still feel young inside can be a daily jolt of misery that causes a lot of stress for many people. It can also lead to worries and stress about unfair ageism in the workplace. Our patients in that demographic know that healthy people generally look better than average, at almost any age. They want to look vibrant but not plumped and stretched with fake faces full of fillers and Botox. By the way, we do use Botox and fillers on our patients. But when done correctly, no one should look like they use them. They should just look fresh and healthy.

They've also learned that you rarely get what you pay for with costly over-the-counter skincare products. I have fond memories of spending several weeks in Singapore with a lovely lady, many years before I met Banding. We went shopping and she gladly forked over $150 an ounce for a small jar of moisturizer. (I can't imagine what it costs now!) I was completely flabbergasted. "How do you know it's any good?" I asked her.

"Because it costs the most," she replied. That was her sole criterion. I didn't want to burst her bubble by telling her she got scammed, because I looked at the fancy label and read the ingredients. I knew that the cream cost only about two dollars to concoct—the rest was for marketing and pure profit. Caveat emptor!

At-Home Treatments

There are many things you can do to keep your skin healthy and glowing.

Stay Out of the Sun!

The most important and easiest thing you can do to protect your skin and your health is to stay out of the sun and use sun protection every day, no matter what your skin tone. Even when it's cloudy or gloomy out—the sun's toxic ultraviolet rays easily penetrate clouds and windows. People who live in the cloudy and rainy Northwest think they're protected, but they aren't—locals are diagnosed with skin cancers more frequently than those in Southern California. Skin cancer rates are skyrocketing around the globe. In 2023, the Netherlands announced a program that offers free dispensers of sunscreen on local beaches because the country's skin cancer rates are at record high levels.

Think of the sun's UVA rays as having an "A" for aging; they alter the DNA in your skin cells and cause skin damage (pigmentation spots, lines, wrinkles, sagging). UVB rays have a "B" for burning. Think of a tan not as something "healthy" but as a low-level burn that over time can develop into one of the three types of skin cancer and even kill you. Why would you want that risk and damage your DNA for a tan?

Basal cell and squamous cell are the most common type of skin cancers. If caught early, they can be removed, and you will be considered cured. (While slow growing, they can kill you if ignored for many years.) Melanoma, like the other two skin cancers, is curable if caught early. If not, it quickly spreads and is often fatal. It can sometimes be hard to detect as the cancerous spot can be extremely small.

Some people use the "But I need my vitamin D!" or "I look so much better with a tan!" excuses to get fried on the beach. Yes, you need sun exposure to trigger vitamin D production. No, you don't have to do that. A daily supplement works just as well.

Look for a broad-spectrum sunscreen with an SPF of 50 that will block UVA and UVB rays. Use a lot of and let it penetrate your skin before you go outside. Reapply every few hours. Avoid products with chemical blockers that are hormone disrupters like oxybenzone. A mineral blocker sunscreen is safer.

Exfoliation

Your skin cells don't live very long. As newer ones are created and push up to the surface from the deeper skin layers, the old, dead ones form the topmost surface of your skin, the stratum corneum. This skin cell turnover in teenage women is about two weeks. In seniors, it can be more than two *months*.

An easy remedy is regular exfoliation to slough off the dead skin cells. You will instantly look refreshed. Men exfoliate automatically when they shave, and women can use gentle exfoliants (not anything harsh, like ground apricot pits) every day or so as part of their regular skincare routine.

High Collagen Foods

Your skin is supported by elastin and collagen fibers that lose elasticity and strength over time. Skincare products containing collagen are useless, because topical collagen can't penetrate to the deeper layers where it's needed. Instead, drink bone broth as often as you can. It's highly nutritious, low in calories, and full of collagen. You can buy it or make it at home by boiling chicken or beef bones. I laugh when I see my wife and her dainty Chinese girlfriends take a boiled chicken foot, stick it in their mouths, move it around, and, somehow, they've removed all the skin and meat and collagen until the only things left are the tiny bones they pop right into their hands. When I've tried to do the same, all I get is a mouthful of gristle!

Progesterone and Estrogen Creams

We prescribe compounded bioidentical progesterone and estrogen creams for almost all of our female patients. While it has a moisturizing effect, the actual function of a progesterone cream is to increase the growth of as well as to strengthen elastin fibers. Over a three- to six-month period, it will also fill in a lot of fine lines and creases, leaving skin smoother. The cream also makes skin thicker and more elastic, so it looks younger. I apply progesterone cream to my face and neck every evening. It not only makes my skin look great, but as a man, I get the added benefit of protection against prostate enlargement.

If this cream is far more effective than anything you can purchase over the counter, why don't dermatologists prescribe it? I wish I knew! Perhaps it's because you're going to be absorbing some progesterone into your system—which you *want* to happen!

Some women also benefit from using an estrogen cream on their faces to make the skin soft and glowing. Facial estrogen cream is not recommended for women with Asian or Mediterranean ancestry, as they tend to get the dark pigmentation areas of melasma, or the "dark mask of pregnancy," caused by high estrogen levels during pregnancy. A high concentration of estrogen in a cream can also cause melasma in those who are genetically prone to develop it.

For men, I often prescribed dilute estradiol cream for those about to have elective surgery. When they apply a thin coating on the incision after it's closed and is healing, the estrogen helps minimize scarring. High testosterone helps men heal faster in their deep tissues, but their skin heals more slowly on the surface because they don't have enough estradiol there. (The skin of post-menopausal women also heals more slowly because they don't have enough estrogen.) I've seen many men who've had their chests cracked for a coronary bypass surgery end up with scars that are almost invisible due to applying estrogen cream to the incision.

An additional benefit to using testosterone, progesterone, and estrogen creams is that bones get thicker. Testosterone stimulates the osteoblasts, the cells that make new bone; estrogens inhibit the activity of osteoclasts, the cells that dissolve old bone; and the progesterone makes the overlying skin soft and flexible. We've done DEXA scans on our female patients and can actually see their bones become thicker as they age instead of thinning out, leading to osteoporosis. Some patients happily tell us they've gone from osteoporosis to osteopenia to normal, strong bones.

What Are Skin Tags?

Skin tags are fleshy little blobs of skin that can appear anywhere on your body, sometimes seemingly overnight. They are more common as you get older. Skin tags are a sign of elevated glucose and insulin resistance. If you see them, have your blood tested as soon as possible to make sure your blood sugar numbers are okay. You can nip off skin tags with scissors or tweezers. If there's a little bleeding, cover the area with a small adhesive bandage for a day or two.

I've heard too many people say, "Oh, I'm prone to skin tags; it's just a genetic thing." Well, it's probably *not* a genetic thing that they're heading toward diabetes. It's far better to reduce insulin resistance so skin tags don't form in the first place.

Medical Treatments

The aesthetic at our spa is to treat patients so they look the best they can for their age. Most of the advanced treatments we do involve the use of lasers.

Fractional Lasers (Fraxel)

A fractional laser ablates small spots on only fractional parts of your skin (hence the name), triggering the growth of new skin. It is an effective procedure that can repair sun damage and remove hyperpigmentation, smooth out texture, and reduce fine lines and wrinkles. There is some downtime after the procedure as the skin peels to reveal new skin growth underneath. You must stay out of the sun for several weeks after treatment. You are doing that already, right?

A word to the wise if you're considering any laser treatments. Any laser is a dangerous device when used by untrained hands. You can get severely burned or have permanent and unsightly pigmentation issues. Many medi-spas or salons offer laser treatments by technicians who have only cursory training and experience. It's legal to do so if a licensed physician is "overseeing" the procedure. Be a savvy consumer and ensure that your treatments are done by experienced personnel.

About Those Annoying Chin Hairs

As women age and female hormone production declines, they'll have more testosterone than estrogen or progesterone. For many women, dark hairs appear on the upper lip or under the chin. The best way to treat them is by getting your sex hormones checked and raising your estrogen and progesterone to decent levels. You can tweeze or wax the hairs for temporary removal, or invest in laser hair removal, which is permanent.

Restore Your Hair

In addition to changes in your skin, changes to your hair over time are visible signs of aging. For the 50 percent of women who have significant hair thinning by age 50, it can be embarrassing and an unwarranted cause for shame, especially for those who consider their hair to be their crowning glory. Wearing a wig every day is uncomfortable. For men who once had a full head of hair, going bald can be equally embarrassing.

Because hair loss is hormonal and genetic, the good news is that it can be treated. We can wake those hair follicles up and make them grow again. Several years ago, we instituted a hair restoration program that has been very successfully regrowing hair in both men and woman.

We don't recommend hair transplants, as that hair will eventually fall out because it was removed from another part of the scalp, and over time that part of the scalp will thin out and take those hairs with it. Hair restoration, on the other hand, prevents loss of the hair you've already got. It is far more cost-effective, less time-consuming, and successful. It starts with a six-month treatment:

- First the nerves to the scalp are blocked so they're totally numb. Next, platelet-rich plasma (PRP), which contains nine growth factors that stimulate hair growth, is drawn from the arms and injected about every centimeter all the way across the scalp. There may be up to 200 small injections going down deep enough to hit the base of the hair follicles. This is repeated three months later.
- Minoxidil (5 percent) is applied during the day. Women are usually told to use the 2 percent version, but the 5 percent product made for men works better and costs less.
- Nizoral shampoo (1 percent active ingredient OTC, 2 percent by prescription) is used at night. It's an anti-fungal, anti-dandruff agent that also stimulates hair growth.
- Every month, micro-needling with PRP is done on the scalp. These needles don't go as deep, so they bring the growth factors to the upper part of the hair follicle.
- After six months, there have been two deep and four superficial applications of the growth factors. We also use a red diode cap to dilate the blood vessels in the scalp and improve the blood flow. You wear it for six minutes once a day, every day, for as long as you want to. We suggest you wear it at least for the first six months.
- Tangible results usually start to appear after about three months. Almost everybody will have some improved growth.
- A touch-up is usually recommended a year or so later.

We are currently experimenting with a diluted rapamycin solution to help trigger both hair growth and stimulation of the stem cells that give hair its darker color. My own hair has been white for a long time, so it is not likely to get darker. But my wife is indeed seeing her salt and pepper hair grow darker. It will be interesting to see how this one turns out. I would love to see a treatment that allowed us to regrow our natural hair color and avoid harsh chemical dyes.

Recommended Supplements for Stress

Refer to Chapter 5 for more details. Discuss the proper doses for your needs as well as any potential contraindications with your doctor before taking any supplements.

Stress Guard/Zen Factor There are limited supplements choices for stress because most things that reduce anxiety will also make you drowsy. We sell Stress Guard in our clinics and Zen Factor through the Relief Factor company. It is made with passionflower for relaxation and a dose of phosphatidyl serine to keep you alert and awake without anxiety.

Chapter 12

The Sleep You Need

Back in our cave-dwelling days, Mother Nature happily watched us pack on the pounds when the weather was warm so we wouldn't die when it got colder. We humans would wake up in the morning and then go out and about doing our daily business—hunting, gathering, farming, fighting, whatever. We'd return to our caves as the sun was going down and the light was changing from white to orange and red.

Those long red wavelengths changed the way our brains functioned by releasing melatonin; the bright daytime sunlight, followed by that dimming light, made us drowsy. As our ancestors sat by the fire, which also had that orange-red glow to it, they ate their evening meal, which stimulated their parasympathetic nervous system to further relax them. They all went to sleep, likely cuddling up together to stay warm, and woke up when the sun rose, or daylight emerged.

Nowadays, there is so much artificial light around us 24/7 that our brains don't know what time of day it actually is. Outdoor light pollution increases every year by 10 percent, according to astronomers, and it's getting harder and harder to see the stars our grandparents could once easily point out. The lamps, energizing blue-lit computer screens, telephones, and televisions in our homes give off brightness long after the sun has set. As it gets later, we yawn, get ready for bed, and flip a switch. It suddenly gets dark, and we tell our bodies it's time to go to sleep. And our bodies say, *What? It was daytime just ten seconds ago! Who do you think you're kidding?*

Poor sleep hygiene is one of the reasons the CDC has estimated that one-third of Americans are sleep-deprived. This is a serious problem. It's not just worrying about nodding off while driving home after work, but sleep deprivation can cause serious health issues.

Why You Need Deep, Replenishing Sleep

How Do You Know You're Getting Enough Sleep?

Everybody's sleep needs are different. Some people are okay with five hours, while others need as much as nine hours. From seven to nine hours seems to be ideal for most of us, although there are people like Albert Einstein who never slept more than four hours a night.

Depending on our internal body clocks, or circadian rhythms, some of us are early birds while others are night owls. My son Jeremy drove us crazy when he was little. He was such a night owl that he stayed be up until the wee hours, then was drowsy and out of it during the day. He was wired differently than the rest of us, and fortunately now has a job where he can set his own hours.

As we age, our sleep needs can change. Some people feel fine with less sleep, while others need much more. A warning sign is if you need much more sleep at night *plus* a daytime nap. If so, you should to be evaluated, as this might be a sign that cognitive alertness is starting to fade. Or, if you usually sleep for a good seven or eight hours and now don't get more than four or five, something is keeping you from getting the deep sleep you need. Get expert medical advice.

The Cycles of Sleep

The Cortisol/Melatonin Cycle

As you read in Chapter 2, your sleep cycle is regulated by the release of the hormone cortisol (it gets you up and energized) and melatonin, the "hormone of darkness" (it gets you ready for sleep). When the cycle is disrupted, sleep is affected. Too much stress, for example, means lots more cortisol floods your body, so it's harder to wind down for the night, while too much light interferes with the release of melatonin.

I recommend avoiding vigorous exercise for three to four hours before bedtime, because it will energize you and make it harder to fall asleep.

The Virtuous Cycle for Sleep

I mentioned the concept of the virtuous cycle in Chapter 1, and there's a particular one for sleep. Deep sleep is when your body produces growth hormone. If you're sleeping well, you're making better growth hormone. If you're making better growth hormone, you're making better muscle. If you're making better muscle, you're making better testosterone. If you're making better muscle and testosterone, you're making brain-derived neurotrophic factors and you're growing your brain and making it healthier and sleeping better.

Health Issues That Can Disrupt Your Sleep

That Annoying Middle-of-the-Night Need to Urinate

When you see ads for adult diapers like Depends, I'll bet you're thinking, *I don't want that to be me.*

Every muscle in your aging body is getting weaker as your anabolic hormone levels decline. That includes the muscles in your bladder, leading to extremely common urination issues as we get older. Yet there is so much unwarranted shame around incontinence that it's rarely brought up in the media in a way that will make you realize there are solutions. A full bladder is going to keep you from getting uninterrupted sleep. If you're getting up more than twice during the night to go to the bathroom, find out what's going on because there will be a reason. Make an appointment with a urologist and get some answers.

For men, it's usually that their enlarged prostate puts pressure on the urethra so the bladder can't empty fully. They might wake up five to seven times a night. An unrecognized side effect of a chronically enlarged bladder is erectile dysfunction. The nerves involved in having an erection travel closely around the bladder. When the bladder is always enlarged, the nerves are stretched and damaged over time. Every young man has had the experience of having an erection with a full morning bladder; that temporary nerve irritation triggered it. Constant, unremitting bladder stretching damages the nerves and inhibits erections in older men. So, if you are getting up multiple times a night, have it checked out before you lose your ability to make love.

For women, whose bladders are usually smaller than men's, spastic bladders are more common. Childbearing will often cause damage to the nerves. As a result, women's bladders start having spasms and there's an urgent need to urinate. Aging bladders don't always fully empty.

There are some medications that relax the bladder. One of them is Botox, which, when injected into the bladder, will numb the spasms for about three months. Anti-cholinergic drugs are often used to make the bladder relax, and they work. But—and this is a big *but*—there is evidence that this class of drugs also accelerates the development of dementia. Talk it over with your doctor if you're prescribed a pill to improve your bladder function.

Sleep Apnea

Sleep apnea is a sleep disorder characterized by irregular breathing. You might not know you have it unless someone sleeping next to you thinks you're dying because you're so quiet and you've stopped breathing for many long seconds. You might be tired all the time and don't know why. Sufferers often snore or snort loudly, gasp for air, and wake up countless times during the night. It's a serious condition that requires treatment.

With age, our carbon dioxide sensing declines, so we have less of a central, or brain stem, drive to trigger our breathing. This can lead to sleep apnea, but the most common cause is an obstruction to your airway, and the primary reason for that is being overweight. There is limited room inside your abdomen, and when you add fat both in and on your belly, the diaphragm is pushed up and breathing becomes restricted and laborious. When you lie down at night, the problem is compounded by the lack of gravity that pulls the fat downward when you are upright.

Additionally, a modest amount of fat is deposited in both the upper and mid-airways, leaving less room for air to pass in and out. At night, when you are asleep, the relaxed muscle tone allows the fat and swelling in your narrowed passageways to close off. Losing weight often helps reduce sleep apnea.

The other major cause of sleep apneas is loss of tone in the facial nerves. This is an age-related neurologic deficit; oral retainers used at night can keep your soft palate from falling into the airway.

Many people use CPAP (continuous positive airway pressure) devices that clear the airway by using pressurized air to push its way through the obstructions. They are noisy and unwieldy, and it can be hard to adjust to having tubes or a mask on your face all night. Surgery is also a possibility; obstructive tissues that are swollen or floppy are fixed so they stay open during sleep. An oral/facial surgeon I know uses a radio-frequency procedure to open the airway for several of our patients who needed this done early in their treatment, before they lost their excess weight.

Digestive Issues

As you read in Chapter 8, eating too close to bedtime or snacking before bed can keep you from losing weight. It can also add to your sleep issues. After you eat, your digestive muscles have to get to work when they should be resting, disrupting your sleep cycle. And, let's face it, that gastrocolic reflex--the need to empty your bowel after eating--disrupts a good night's sleep more than a full bladder would. Don't worry about going to bed without your bedtime snack. Your body actually gets better rest without it.

Hormone Deficiencies

Several of the most common complaints from women during perimenopause and menopause are insomnia, chronically interrupted sleep, and night sweats. Supplementation of testosterone can help you make more of your own estrogen, or testosterone and estrogen together might be recommended when indicated. Progesterone can also be recommended as it has pronounced sedative effects.

I apply a potent, prescription progesterone cream to my face and neck every evening to get both the sedative, sleep-promoting effect, and smoother, less-wrinkled skin. (Yes, I am every bit as vain as my wife. And given that I am 30 years her senior, I need more of the skin-enhancing effects that progesterone provides!)

How to Improve Your Sleep Hygiene

Set Up a Nightly Sleep Routine and Stick to It

If you had a baby, I'm sure you had a nightly bedtime routine—bath, books, lullabies—to put the infant to sleep. I'll also bet that you continued with a sleep routine to get your toddler and older child to sleep, too.

Sleep hygiene is all about creating a nightly routine for yourself that will train your brain to slow you down and get you ready for bed. What you want to try to do is re-create, as closely as possible, that scenario of our cave-dwelling ancestors when they returned home as the sun was setting, had a meal, talked and wound down, then snuggled up against another warm body and fell asleep in the dark. When your bedroom becomes your personal haven of relaxation, it will also be a trigger for a good night's sleep.

You want minimal stress, minimal anxiety, and minimal stimulation at night. (Easier said than done!) Try to stick to your routine whenever possible. These tips will help:

- Allow darkness to come on gradually. Start dimming your lights at least one hour before bedtime. If you are fortunate enough to have a fireplace in your bedroom, the orange light of the fire (similar to sunset) will trigger the release of melatonin. Use incandescent or LED light bulbs if possible. A rheostat to dim them tends to shift the color to an orange shade. The color shift and dimmer light both prepare you for sleep.

- Watching relaxing entertainment is fine, but avoid the late evening news or any kind of upsetting movie. These will cause adrenaline and cortisol surges that will keep you jittery and leave you wide awake.

- Turn off all electronic devices that emit brain-stimulating blue light at least one hour before bedtime. You want dim red or orange light, not bright white or blue. Using a blue-light filter on your computer screen or other devices can also help.
- Do a few gentle stretches or some yoga poses. Yoga nidra uses meditation and is especially helpful for pre-sleep relaxation.
- Listen to soft, soothing music, preferably without lyrics.
- Read a printed book (not on devices like Kindles—save those for daytime reading) that won't be too stimulating.
- Take a hot shower or bath or drink a cup of hot herbal tea. Heat relaxes your muscles and lowers your blood pressure. Soaking in a tub with magnesium-rich Epsom salts also soothes achy muscles.
- Cuddling in bed with a warm body is helpful. If you don't have a partner, a cat or a dog will do fine. The warmth of a person or a pet next to your body is akin to those primal needs of cave dwellers—they snuggled together for survival and warmth as the fire died down during the night. If you're able to modify your lifestyle to more closely re-create the conditions we were evolved to be in, you will sleep more naturally.
- If you still have trouble sleeping, talk to your doctor about trying any of the supplements listed on page 274.

My Nighttime Sleep Routine

During the evening at home, I've programmed the lights so that one comes on in the living room when the rest of the house is dark. Banding and I have already taken our evening walk. We cuddle on the sofa, and she puts her head on my shoulder while we talk gently.

Once Ivory takes her shower, I tuck her in, give her a good night hug, and tell her how much she's loved. She snuggles down with her cat. I go upstairs, take my shower, and take my sleepy-time supplements.

Banding and I get into bed, and I sit with my back against the headboard. She sits between my legs with her back against me. I put my arms around her, and we watch a calming video or just talk and eventually she falls asleep on my chest. We do this every night. I'm always so grateful that she feels so safe and secure that she drifts off in my arms and on my chest. I turn off the TV, lay her down gently, and in a few minutes, I'm also fast asleep.

Power Naps Can Give You Power

Nappers are like night owls. You either are or you aren't! I know people who can never nap even when they're keeling over with exhaustion. If I find I'm tired after lunch, I'll set a timer on my phone for 20 to 30 minutes for a quick nap. To get the benefits of a daytime nap, you want to sleep for at least 20 minutes but not more than 30. This will help you recover your energy without being groggy from the nap. Sleeping more than 30 minutes lets you drop into a deeper sleep that is harder to wake up from.

If you need a nap, it's not an indulgence. But as I said previously, if you find yourself needing more naps than usual, see a doctor. If you are sedentary and don't have a lot of muscle strength, napping can make you more tired. Strong muscles don't fatigue.

As an aside, a good boss is going to realize that sometimes employees need a nap—and that will boost productivity if they let them take one. On the other end, most hard-working young people get brain fog from sitting and staring at a computer screen for hours on end. For many of them, it's not a nap they need, it's a little exercise. My employees' salaries are based on their productivity, so I don't closely monitor their hours. I wish more employees were treated this way. In some companies, workers feel the need to eat sugary donuts or chocolate chip cookies at 3 p.m. to stay awake. (My employees' needs are paramount to me and to the success of my clinics. I suspect my obsession with happy staff and stable families is, in part, an expression of my guilt for never being there for my first family, and I don't want to be responsible for doing that with my staff. When I tell employees that their families come first, I mean it.)

Avoid Prescription Sleeping Pills

When I was a country doctor, I went to the hospital for morning rounds one day and found the nurses upset. One of my doctor colleagues had called in at two in the morning and changed the orders for all his hospitalized patients. When he came in the next morning to make his rounds, he did not remember calling and changing the orders. He became furious and demanded that they all be changed back. It turned out that he was prescribed Ambien by *his* doctor. Ambien is one of the most frequently prescribed drugs for sleep disorders. Under its influence, my colleague got retrograde amnesia and had no memory of what he'd done, which is common with this medication. The nurses filed a complaint, and when he was told to list his medications, hospital authorities realized what had happened. He was *mortified*. He was also lucky that he wasn't suspended and that nobody died or was harmed because he took a pill to help him sleep.

Many other prescription sleep meds have similar or problematic side effects. Worse, they put you in artificial sleep and prevent you from getting the natural, deep sleep you need. Instead, you are drugged into unconsciousness, and because you aren't refreshed, you become more exhausted, so you take more meds. This can start an anti-virtuous cycle.

Almost nobody needs these meds. There are far better ways for most people who have trouble sleeping to get the rest they need. Speak to your doctor about trying a natural supplement before you take them.

Recommended Supplements for Sleep

Refer to Chapter 5 for more details. Discuss the proper doses for your needs as well as any potential contraindications with your doctor before taking any supplements.

If you're having difficulties sleeping, try some of the tips in the sleep hygiene section above. It may take days or weeks before you can change your sleeping pattern.

You might have heard about CBD, the non-psychoactive compound in cannabis, as a sleep aid (THC is the primary psychoactive compound that gets you high). I don't recommend smoking, vaping, or chewing gummies with CBD because we don't know what the long-term effects might be. There is a widespread assumption that the much higher incidence of psychosis we are seeing in cannabis users is being triggered by the THC, and the marketing being done for the CBD compounds made from hemp is based on the unproven conjecture that they're safe due to the lack of THC. Don't self-medicate with assumptions. Wait for long-term, peer-reviewed studies before using CBD.

I don't advise mixing sleep supplements since I do not have reliable research on most of them when used in combination.

Melatonin The melatonin we make for our patients comes in 1-, 2-, 3-, 5-, and 10-mg strengths. In our clinic, we start with 1 mg at bedtime each night for three or four nights, then increase the dose by 1 mg every three or four nights until the patient is sleeping soundly with pleasant dreams. If you take too much melatonin, your dreams will become so vivid that they will disrupt your sleep. If that happens, reduce your dose to the lowest and then increase it again very slowly.

Those who can tolerate higher levels of melatonin, doses over 10 mg/night, might find that it triggers increased human growth hormone release. This can help you grow new tissue, which can be of significant benefit in healing as well as increase strength and endurance. Some oncologists use very high doses, up to 40 mg two to three times daily, to help a patient's immune system fight cancers.

Make sure your supplement is from a reputable company. A recent study published online at the JAMA Network showed that a whopping 22 of the 25 different melatonin brands they investigated were mislabeled. The amount of melatonin varied considerably from the stated amount.

L-Theanine L-theanine is the compound in green tea with a sedative effect. It can help mellow you out and reduce anxiety. Instead of drinking multiple cups of tea, which can have a diuretic effect, a supplement might be worth a try. We carry one in our online store, and many of our patients use it for relaxation and sleep. You can get the same effects with a cup or two of green tea, but the pills work faster.

Valerian Even the ancient Greeks and Romans were familiar with the relaxing properties of this plant, which is why it's been used to treat insomnia for centuries. It's also used for anxiety, depression, and to treat hormonal symptoms of perimenopause and menopause.

Z Factor Full disclosure: I developed this pill due to patient demand and sell it nationally at relieffactor.com. We named it Z as in the ZZZs you get while sleeping! It contains a tiny bit of melatonin; a big dose of L-theanine, the sedative component of green tea; and GABA, a neurotransmitter that damps down brain activity. Most people fall into a deep sleep within 15 minutes of taking it. If you tend to wake up at two in the morning, you might need to take two before bedtime. My wife takes one every night, and I usually take two. I know a few folks who use three each night. Remember Rule #2: The proper dose of anything is enough to do the job.

Chapter 13

Passion and Purpose

My mother was born and raised in a log cabin without electricity or running water. Her parents couldn't afford a horse or mule or wagon, so the family either walked or used an ox cart that looked like something out of the Middle Ages. (Their slow and reliable ox was not as fast or fancy as the horse or mule the neighbors had, but it was "strong as an ox.") She never went to college, but worked all her life as a civil service stenographer. She and my dad raised me to be as fiercely independent as they were, as well as inquisitive and unafraid of life and its challenges. They weren't rich or famous. They weren't well-educated and had no social advantages. But they both took on the world on their own terms and came out laughing. I never saw either of my parents discouraged by life.

When Mom was 79, my stepfather died. She mourned for a year or two, and then when she was 81, she declared that she wanted to see many of the current Seven Wonders of the World, and off she went. She stayed in a monastery in Peru to visit Machu Picchu, took a *felucca* down the Nile and rode camels at the pyramids of Giza, climbed the Eiffel Tower, and took a long dusty hike to the ruins in Petra. A year later, she decided she wanted to set foot on every continent, and traveled to Asia, Europe, and Australia. She even took a ship to the South Pole to see the penguins on the Ross Ice Shelf. Two years after that, she decided to explore South Korea, so she went there for two months. At 84, she sailed the seven seas by booking a four-month around-the-world cruise. That one was so much fun that she did it twice in three years. Her only complaint was the number of old men hitting on her during the cruises. "Those old guys want a nurse, not a wife," she told me.

She enjoyed every day she had allotted to her. When she wanted to do something, she got it done. She took up oil painting and dance and went to the gym five days a week. I treated her at my clinic for the last 23 years of her life. I was overjoyed to see her exuberance when her hormone levels returned to those of a much younger woman. She followed a healthy diet, and her days and nights were filled with activities.

When Mom was 88, she called me on her Life Alert ("I've fallen and I can't get up . . . ") button when she got lost going to the gym, as I wrote about in Chapter 7. I couldn't help looking back and wondering if that episode was the beginning of what would cause her death two years later. She got lost again at 90, but this time she was confused. I sent her to the hospital, and they discovered five brain tumors. As the end approached, her only comment on dying was, "This waiting around to die is the horse's patoot!" I never saw her afraid or depressed. She died in my arms five months later. I held her as she passed with my cheek touching hers so she would know that she was not alone and was loved as she left this world for the next.

She lived while she was alive. You might not want to sail down the Nile or hike in Jordanian deserts, but I want you to have the passion and purpose in your life that my mom did.

Living Your Purpose

Steve Douglas is a friend I've known since high school. We joined the military together. He was an accomplished pilot who was shot down three times in Vietnam. Every time he was recuperating from his injuries, he insisted on returning to Vietnam if they trained him on a different aircraft. They did. He knew his purpose, and nothing was going to stop him from fulfilling it. He was some role model!

No matter how old you are, you need a reason to get up in the morning so you can do something that's rewarding. If you're still vigorous, I'll bet you're still working at something. Not necessarily at a job, but at something that engages you. At 76, I still work full-time and am having a great time. I have no intention of retiring—but if I did, I'd want to be just like my mother. In fact, I'm looking to grow my companies and maybe start a few new ones. I don't want to fall into the retirement trap—while ending your professional career can be a well-deserved reward for decades of hard work, the abrupt change to a regular schedule can trigger anxiety, depression, and inertia. Something my mom was determined never to happen to her. I believe one of the reasons people become shells of their former selves with retirement and beyond is that in large measure their hormone loss kills their sense of purpose.

Part of what longevity's about is finding a team to support you through all your years. If you feel that you have nothing to live for, how did you arrive at that place? What needs aren't being fulfilled? Who can you turn to for help?

Since I am a poster child for reinvention, I can tell you that it is possible for a do-over at any age. For the first part of my life, I was a student and a soldier. The soldier convinced me I wanted to be a physician. I became a student again and then a physician. I was a country doctor for 20 years, and when I became Fat Jerry I could hear Mother Nature cackling in the background. That spurred me to become a longevity doctor, expanding from one clinic to three. Then, as you know by now, my supplement business took off, and after realizing that when people feel better, they want to look better, I added the medical spa business. My next challenge is taking all of the businesses national. After that, who knows. Ask me in 10 or 15 years when I'm 85 or 90 and I might have a few new businesses in the works!

What drives me is loving what I do. Like Reed Carruthers, who's in charge of the fulfillment center—he doesn't call it a warehouse—for our supplements. He runs that place so that our employees also love what they do because they know they're important. I love it when he asks me to come over to talk to them. "Let me explain something to you," I tell everyone. "You might think you just work in a warehouse, but without you, all the work by the executive staff, the marketing people, the radio and TV hosts that tell people about the products, all of that would be worthless, because nothing would ever get to the people who wanted it. It's all because of you.

You, ladies and gentlemen, are the ones shipping countless packages every day to the people who need them." Then I give them my heartfelt thanks for their hard work. I pay them well and respect every one of them. Without them, I would not have a supplement business.

Use Your Strengths/Minimize Your Weaknesses

Some of us are strong, fast, and have great endurance, while others are church mice, content to sit in the back and watch others run races. You are what you are. Acknowledge your strengths; minimize your weaknesses. Too many of us minimize our strengths, the things we're good at. We don't think they're important or valuable because they're easy for us. Instead, we harp on what we *can't* do. Be smart enough to know what your flaws are so that you can address them. There should never be any shame about asking for help if you need it. My success has not been earned by just my own work. I have an incredible team of people around me, and every one does their job better than I ever could. My partners, Lynn Kasel and Robert Wagner, have skill sets that, frankly, leave me awestruck. I know the physiology and biochemistry; they understand finance and business far better than I could ever hope to.

When you maximize your strengths and use them for both your own and other people's benefit, the results will be positive, even if they aren't exactly what you'd planned. For example, my ability to create an effective system to improve longevity was something I discounted for a long time. Learning and teaching others about longevity took time and was difficult, but for some reason I didn't see it as anything special, when it was! I've since come to recognize that part of why people pay attention to me and keep calling my radio show is that I can take their complex biochemistry issues and make them easy to understand.

For instance, no one really cares to know how much aromatase is present in abdominal fat, or that the testosterone molecule differs from estradiol, the primary human estrogen, in one hydroxyl group. Instead, I clearly explain that one of the reasons people get weak and fatigued as they gain weight is that their belly fat is turning their testosterone into estrogen. Losing muscle, along with a fading sex drive and ambition, is due to their dropping testosterone and rising estrogen levels. It also puts the increased risk of erectile dysfunction in focus since that condition increases in proportion to the expansion of a man's abdominal girth. *That* gets a man's attention.

"Love thy neighbor as thyself" is one tenet of Judeo-Christian scripture that I think is widely misunderstood. It doesn't say love thy neighbor *instead* of yourself. It presumes that you love yourself *first*. You must take care of yourself *first*. You can't love other people if you don't love yourself. Love yourself so that you are truly able to love your neighbor. You were made to be that unique individual, you. Embrace yourself and accept your unique value.

Loving yourself also means being honest with yourself about who you really are and what you really want. It takes a lot of courage to do that—but it's never too late to try. I made a mistake getting married the first time. It took me decades to be honest with my wife, who was an incredible woman and mother and deserved so much better. When I reached the point where I was so unhappy that I could not bear to live half a life any longer, I finally told her, "Sweetheart, it's not you. You are a wonderful human being and wife, and you've done nothing wrong. I've just never been happy being married from day one. There's no way for you to make me happy." She was deeply hurt, and I was deeply ashamed and pained, knowing I'd hurt her. But when she fell in love with someone else, she was able to be brutally honest with me, too. "I never really knew tenderness and love until I met John," she told me. I couldn't possibly get upset at hearing that because it was true. I told her how sorry I was that I couldn't give that to her, and we both moved on, happier people who remain friends and celebrate the children we created together.

It's easier to be positive about your future when you feel strong and healthy. It's hard to plan for anything when you're in pain, or don't have the energy to shop for groceries or get the mail. When you sleep well, you're producing the growth hormone that allows you to grow new tissue and repair those worn-out joints . . . so you can be more physically active . . . so you can make even more muscle and get even stronger . . . so you will have you even more energy. The virtuous cycle we need is all connected.

Deal with Envy and Regrets

My patients spend a lot of time in our clinics, and over the years they confide in me or the other doctors about their hopes, fears, joy, and heartaches. Similar themes come from the callers to my radio show. Many callers talk about regrets—what they could or should have done when they were younger, and how they fear they are running out of time. When their health and stamina improve, and depression and anxiety lessen, they are better able to create an action plan to push past the memories of what could-have-been and concentrate on the what's-coming-next instead.

Find the Antidote to the Poison of Regrets

When you turn 50 and realize your life is more than half over, it's assessment time. Where are you now? Where do you want to be? What have you not done yet? This is all part of assessing your longevity, because if you don't have a good reason to get out of bed in the morning, you're not going to get up.

I doubt there is anyone reading this book who doesn't have some regrets about things done or not done in life. Or not done as well as they could or should have. Yet regrets will age your psyche like the sun will age your skin. Your cortisol levels go up as immune response goes down. Guilt, regrets, and depression are killers.

My biggest regret is that I was not there for my children of my first marriage. I was rarely home. When I was, I was too exhausted to give them the emotional support and guidance they needed and deserved. I know I can never undo the damage done to them. I now spend a lot of time with my daughter Ivory because I know what I did wrong the first time. I could poison myself with regrets, but I do know that I got married because it seemed like I couldn't have done anything else at the time. I was only 20 and unable to voice what I knew in my heart was wrong. If I'd known then what I know now, the trajectory of my life would have been very different.

Most people do the best they know how at any given point in their lives. One of the most important things we can do is forgive ourselves. If you're human, you're going to make mistakes. There's no way around that. The questions shouldn't be, "Am I going to make mistakes?" but

"How do I compensate for my screwups? How do I make restitution to those I've harmed if restitution is possible?" Frequently, it's not. When it is not, the task is to recognize reality and move on.

As Omar Khayyam said, "The finger of fate writes; and, having writ, moves on." We need to do the same thing. Write this chapter of your life and move on. Regrets are not productive unless they spur you on to do something that you otherwise would not have. Regrets for the sake of regrets lead you down into the gully of guilt . . . where sometimes you can no longer find the path to lead you up and out.

Pencils have erasers; lives don't. We're writing with indelible ink. If there are extra marks on the paper, so be it. Forgive yourself for being human. Letting go of an unchangeable past can be an insurmountable task. Some spend their later years torturing themselves with regrets and negative emotions. I hope that won't be you.

Don't Let Yourself Become Your Parents (Unless They Were Your Role Models for What Is Good in Life)

Patients tell me a lot of personal details. One of the most common laments is, "Ohmigod, I'm turning into my mother/father!" If your parents were attentive, nurturing, and like the kind of person you'd like to be, of course you want to act the same way. In my experience, I find it deeply saddening to hear more negatives about family situations than positives. But it's never too late to identify negative behaviors so you can become better aware of any hurtful patterns and confront them.

Banding's upbringing was dire; her father beat her, and her mother showed her little affection. Her parents married because the party boss at the factory where her father worked as the company doctor decided they would make a good couple. They were never in love or compatible but had a child because the government told them to. The one-child-to-a-family policy was in place. When their daughter was born in Chengdu, her disappointed father named her Banding—a name which means half boy, because in China at the time the assumption was that a girl was only half as good as a boy. (Chinese girls are usually given descriptive names like Soft Breeze or Blossoming Flower.) He told her she would never amount to anything. She was determined to prove him wrong. She worked several jobs to save up enough money to leave China and find a better and more fulfilling life. For Banding, freedom is critical to her happiness. She loves her adopted America with a passion that I wish more native-born Americans shared. When Banding became a mother, her harsh upbringing and approach to child-rearing have been something she's had to work on. She doesn't want her difficult relationship with her parents to be what Ivory has with her.

In our home, Banding rules as the Chinese Tiger Mom, and she can't help comparing herself and Ivory to the other Chinese Tiger Moms of her acquaintance and their children. When the brilliant son of a friend of ours, who was finishing tenth grade, started getting recruitment letters from multiple Ivy League schools, which pretty much guarantees he'll get in anywhere he chooses, Banding's response was, "Nobody's sending letters to *our* daughter." I said, "Honey, she's in *fifth* grade. Would you relax?" Banding was taught to expect near-perfection, and my job as the older, mellowed, and experienced dad is to dampen that down a bit. Ivory is a name Banding chose because ivory is rare, pale, and valuable, like our hybrid daughter. Ivory will respond far better to hugs, love, and encouragement than she will to demands. Ivory is lucky that Banding and I are both fiercely independent, showing her the importance of working hard, traveling the world, and engaging with all kinds of people.

Envy is like regrets. Social media has distorted what we think other people have because they're showing off vacation snaps on a tropical beach or those perfect at-home shots. We don't know what goes on behind closed doors. What you think is a golden reality is probably something you'd never want for yourself.

Passion, Joy, Love, Gratitude, and Longevity

Keeping passion and joy in your life should be one of your top priorities as you get older.

This might sound corny, but when I go outside for my morning jog, gazing out over the lake, with the trees surrounding me and the mountains in the distance, I'm incredibly grateful to be alive at that moment.

Even when the wind is cold and the rain is pelting down, I relish what is before me.

Before I met Banding, I thought I would never marry again, because I was married to medicine. I didn't lack for friends, lovers, or travel companions. Yet we quickly started to mesh and realized that her needs were my strengths, and my needs were her strengths. We decided to spend the rest of our lives together. I have a partner who loves me and trusts me, and I am especially grateful to have been given a second chance at love.

Some of my religious friends consider me a bit of a heathen because I don't share their religious convictions. But if talking to God constitutes prayer, I chat with Him several times a day, although my prayers consist of simple but heartfelt thank you's. I have been blessed with so much in my life that for me to ask God for anything more would be sheer greed. (I do ask for help for my employees or friends who are having difficulties in their lives. But since those prayers are not for me, I don't feel bad asking.) I've got it all. Yes, I'm old, but I'm healthy, and productive and I love every aspect of my life. Except for the inevitable problems and stresses that pop up, or saying goodbye to loved ones whose time has come.

I've learned that what I once thought was a must-have is not important anymore. That's a gift you can give yourself. My mother gave me this sage advice many years ago:

"Jerry," she said, "nobody's ever going to care about you as much as you do. People just don't give a damn. They're busy running their own lives. So why are you worried about what they think about you when they're not even thinking about you? Go live your own life."

Richard Tonelli's Rules of Life

Here's my patient Richard once again, on his rules for living:

After 20 years as a patient with Dr. Mixon and the Longevity Medical Clinic, my philosophy of life became: To Live, to Love, to Learn, and to Leave a Legacy. It's the Living part that I want to address:

- Be kind to yourself.
- Sleep so your body can repair itself.
- Eat to nourish your body and brain.
- Exercise to build muscle and stamina.
- Exercise your brain to think and discuss.
- Use time effectively by prioritizing primary goals and writing them down. Make lists of daily tasks.
- Enjoy the journey of life.
- Be kind to others.
- Don't forget to laugh. A lot.

A Few Words About My Dad

I started this chapter writing about my mom, so let me end it with my dad.

My dad quit school in the eighth grade because his father died, and as the oldest son he had to earn money to support his mom and siblings. He plowed other people's fields with a mule and hand plow for 50 cents a day. My dad joined the Navy when he was 18. He was 28 when he married my mom, who was 16. I was born when she was 17. She and I kind of grew up together. Dad and Mom divorced when I was 21.

Dad left the Navy after 31 years and became a carpenter and construction worker, remaining fit and active as much as he could. He settled down in Texas and grew pecans in the front yard and gardened in the back. When he was in his 80s, he totaled three cars in less than a year. It was only luck that he didn't kill someone. Even though he was legally blind, he refused to stop driving. During his last hospital stay, I called his doctor and asked him to please report my dad to the DMV so they could yank his license. The doctor laughed. "I wish," he said, "but this is Texas, and if a driver can hold their white cane out the window and feel the bumps in the middle of the road, they're safe to drive."

My dad kept driving until he had a surprise visitor one day. After his second wife died, the woman who'd been his teenage girlfriend—before he joined the Navy and married my mother—found out that he was single again. She flew from South Carolina to San Angelo, showed up at his front door, and said, "I'm not gonna miss another chance. I'm here and I'm staying." They got married, and when my dad couldn't garden any longer, they moved to a small house in the Carolinas next to her kids and grandkids, about half a mile from where my dad grew up on his family farm. One of my sons built them a ramp for their wheelchairs. May, bless her, took away his car keys, and gave his car to her kids who lived nearby. They happily lived their last years together. I placed him in a nursing home only when the end was near, and he needed round-the-clock care. Even in his last few weeks, Dad was a bit of a rogue. I went to visit him one day and the nurse said, "Your old man would make a pass at a fence post if I put a dress on it!" Talk about libido—and longevity!

May died a few weeks after Dad. They missed their chance to be together as teenagers, but shared their last several years on earth, and from what I could see, adored one another.

When my father was near death, he told me what he wanted on his tombstone. It was as simple and honest as he was. The inscription reads: "He did his best."

I hope that when I leave this world, my own epitaph will be the same.

Recommended Supplement for Passion and Purpose

Refer to Chapter 5 for more details. Discuss the proper doses for your needs as well as any potential contraindications with your doctor before taking any supplements.

Taurine The only supplement that has some data backing it up to show extended health and life span is taurine, which cells use to produce energy. I estimate that the 1,500 mg I take daily will be effective.

A Few Final Thoughts . . .

Not long ago, three people who called in to my Saturday radio show all had the same thing in common. They were over 75 and their doctors were not being aggressive with their care—not even ordering any tests anymore. Simply because they were old, and it wasn't cost-effective to take care of them. I got a little steamed and said to each one of them, "You know what? You need a new doctor. What a jerk!" The callers laughed, which reminded me of this old canard, which I was only too happy to tell them: If you go to the Naval Academy in Annapolis, the lowest person in the graduating class is referred to as the anchor. If you go to West Point, the lowest graduating cadet is called the goat. If you go to any medical school in this country, the lowest graduating student in the class is called a *doctor*.

You have learned by now that being old and feeling old are not the same thing. Aging is not a disease. It's the normal *ha-ha-I'm-still here* rebuttal to Mother Nature. The fact that we will all live longer now is one of the great gifts of science. We are one of the first generations that gets to decide what to do with this knowledge, and to strive for the kind of longevity we want to have. The kind that warrants thinking outside the box and realizing that the doomsayers in the medical profession might not understand that there are many, many things you can do to improve your longevity.

When I was told I was 90 percent disabled, I was only 21. I could have wallowed. I could have given up like so many of my fellow soldiers did.

Instead, I was determined to become a healer rather than a killer. The first turning point arrived when I became a doctor. The second arrived when I was a middle-aged 50-year-old and knew I was on that slippery slope down to where Mother Nature wanted me, six feet under. Twenty-six years later, I am much stronger, faster, leaner, smarter, and my wife swears I am sexier than I was at 50. Despite my disability and the challenges that have come as years go by, I have gone from exhausted and depressed Fat Jerry to living a vigorous, energetic life full of joy, love, strength, and insights, thanks to the tools and strategies I have used to take control of my health that you've read about in this book.

The biochemistry of your body is complex, but the things we need to do to kick that biochemistry into gear are pretty simple. Whether you are an urban apartment dweller, a suburban homeowner, or living in the country, you can go outside and enjoy your surroundings on a walk. Wherever you go and whatever your pace, you'll still burn those calories. You'll get stronger. You'll feel better. You'll feel empowered. You'll have clicked into that virtuous cycle where every step you take is better than the one before.

The innovative medical practice I've pioneered empowers people to take control of their aging and live their best lives. We've got a saying in our clinics that if you don't like what time and gravity are doing to you, come see us, we can help. But if you reach the point that you no longer care, we can't. You must care enough about yourself to make changes in your life. I know you are worth the effort. The question is, do you?

It is my fervent hope that you have gained a new perspective on what it means to age gracefully and discover the practical steps you can take to improve your own health, well-being, and longevity no matter how old you are.

Here's to your happy and healthy long life!

Acknowledgments

My thanks to the many people who have worked together to bring this book into existence.

Madeleine Morel, the agent who put together an amazing team to guide me through this process. Karen Moline, a fine writer who was able to take my disjointed and disorganized ramblings and convert them into coherent and, I hope, enjoyable chapters. Without her talent and corrections I would have never gotten to completion. Dee Dee DeBartlo, our project manager, who pushed, nagged, and cajoled the entire team, mostly me, into meeting deadlines and goals. Harriet Bell, my super-savvy line editor. Deri Reed, my eagle-eyed copy editor. Sibylle Kazeroid, my extremely thorough proofreader.

Then there's our jacket designer, David Gee, who worked to make the prose into an attractive package, Deborah Feingold, the photographer whose camera skills allowed me to be shown at my best despite my age and old injuries, and the amazingly talented and efficient team at Mayfly Design, especially Jess LaGreca for her superb work on the book's interior.

Then come the folks who make my life the kind of joy that allows me the energy and leisure to do the book. Banding, my wife of 19 years and the greatest joy in my life. I swear she should give wife lessons to all the disaffected, disgruntled women out there who are killing their souls trying to have it all. No one has it all! This brave, adventurous woman, whose youthful adventures and world explorations captured my heart two decades ago, made a conscious choice to rebuild her life around me and our daughter Ivory. I, in turn, try every day of my life to make her the happiest woman on the planet, and to help Ivory become the kind of brave, knowledgeable woman who has the ability to mold her own life into whatever form she chooses to give her fulfilment and joy.

Lynn Kasel and Bob Wagner, the intelligent and skilled guys who serve as my company president and CFO respectively. It is their skills, knowledge, and good judgment that give me the financial success I enjoy. It is a wonderful arrangement; they do 90 percent of the work and I take 90 percent of the credit. It is their brilliance that allows me the leisure to spend four to five hours a day reading medical journals and learning about human aging so that I can transmit the new things I learn to the doctors who see the patients, and make videos for patients as well as the public television special that triggered the production of this book. Reed Caruthers who runs our company fulfillment center is a joy. His skill and hard work get the products we sell to the people who need them to enhance their lives.

Speaking of public television, Jerry Adams and Dennis Allen shepherded me through the production and performance for the 90-minute fundraiser for public television. Two real pros who took a rookie under their wing and let me soar.

The doctors at Longevity Medical Clinics who actually see the patients, and who work hard every day to make our patients stronger, faster, leaner, smarter, sexier, and happier. You ladies and gentlemen are the backbone of the clinics. Thank you one and all for joining me. And Samira Ummat, you did indeed put on your Big Girl Pants and became a fine medical director. It is a delight working with you and watching you become better and better at what you do.

To my first and long-ago grown-up family. That I did not do a better job of being a father and husband in those long-ago decades is my one enduring regret in life.

Finally, but not least, to my patients, past and present. That you have trusted me with the opportunity to help you with your myriad issues humbles me. I do and have done my best to live up to the honor and trust you placed in me. I do not always know the answers, but I do my best to find out when your questions reveal my limitations. Thank you for making me learn new things every day of my life.

I am truly blessed by all of you!

Jerry N. Mixon, MD

Why You Need a Longevity Physician—and What You Will Find at Longevity Medical Clinics

There are three very good reasons a longevity physician is needed to treat your aging issues.

1. Let me ask you this question: If you were suffering from chest pains and thought you might be having a heart attack, would you call your son's pediatrician to help? Obviously, the answer is no—the reason being that you do not expect a pediatrician to have the knowledge base and experience needed to treat a dangerous cardiac problem in an adult. Nor would you consult a psychiatrist for your obstetrical issues or an orthopedic surgeon for a facelift.

   Medicine has grown so complex that we have divided our care into areas of specialization. Longevity medicine is a new but very legitimate area of care. No other physician has the specialized body of knowledge needed to know which tests need to be run, how to interpret those tests based not on "normal," which is what other specialties do, but rather on optimal for you as an individual. Longevity physicians also utilize therapies that are often a bit unorthodox but can be very effective for improving your quality of life.

2. The second issue is cost and payment. Most medical clinics and physicians are dependent on insurance coverage for their reimbursement. But aging is not a disease! Getting older is a natural and normal process. Growing slower, weaker, and less capable, both mentally and physically, is a normal part of the aging process. But as a consequence of aging not constituting a disease, its treatment is not considered to be necessary, and hence is not covered by insurance. When people ask me why my clinics do not accept their insurance, I point out that they have it backwards; their insurance does not cover aging, because aging is not a disease. On the other hand, I believe that anything that eventually kills 100 percent of its victims deserves to be treated aggressively!

3. The third reason your family doctor cannot address this problem effectively is *time*. The average physician visit is now about six to seven minutes of face-to-face time with the patient. Yes, you might be in your doctor's clinic for a long time during your visit, but most of that is spent seeing people other than the actual physician.

   At Longevity Medical Clinics our physicians spend at least an hour with the patient at every visit. The aging process is complex. It is not the result of just one or two factors. So we need the time to go over extensive laboratory work and well as detailed evaluation of how you are responding clinically to our multifaceted interventions. That simply cannot be rushed. The single most common complaint I hear from my physicians is that even though they have an hour scheduled for each patient visit, they often feel that they run short of time.

What Happens When You Come to a Longevity Medical Clinic

The initial evaluation will involve the familiar forms and questionnaires. We need to collect a comprehensive history of your health and medical problems. But equally important, we want to know a great deal of detail about how well, or poorly, you are functioning in your day-to-day life. You might be completely "normal." But as we say, normal is great at 18, but by 50 "normal" stinks. And it gets worse every year after that.

We will take the standard vitals of your blood pressure, weight, pulse, and temperature. We will also measure your body fat and muscle mass in each arm, leg, and, most critically, in your torso. I hope you understand by now that fat and muscle are both highly active producers of hormones, peptides, cytokines, and immune factors that have strongly opposing effects on your health and longevity.

A patient's laboratory report averages about 70 pages and will include tests that your primary care physician has likely never run for their patients. It includes genetic factors, inflammatory markers, eight different hormone levels, and specialized tests to determine how tough life has been on your overall system up to this point. Putting this information together with your medical history as well as your personal goals for the clinic will allow your doctor to design a program specifically for you as an individual.

Your Longevity Medical Clinic doctor will prescribe medications and hormones to address any systemic deficiencies as shown by the lab work. They will also prescribe supplements designed to address medical and clinical issues above and beyond those addressed by the prescription medications. From our point of view, anything that alters how your body functions is effectively a drug whether or not the FDA considers it to be so. We do not want you taking supplements just because a friend or an ad you came across made claims for its use. Many of the medications prescribed will be compounded by a specialized pharmacy to the specifications your doctor has created just for you.

Two weeks after you start the program, you will get a follow-up call to check on you. Four weeks after that, your entire laboratory panel will be repeated. The doctor will compare your current values with those you initially had, and adjust your medications and supplements based on your progress and the lab changes. Again, during your hour-long visit, your doctor will be looking closely at how you are feeling and functioning, and any new issues will be addressed.

This process will be repeated in another two months, and again every three months for the first two or three years. Once we know you are doing well and are stable, the visits might be stretched out to every four months instead of every three. The reason for this is simple. Life will continue to have it ups and downs and unexpected occurrences. Besides, you are still growing a bit older all the time, so your needs will evolve; that, in turn, will impact the interventions we need to make you as strong, fast, lean, smart, and sexy as humanly possible at any age.

I have been on my longevity therapy for 26 years now. I continue to get periodic blood draws and my physician at Longevity continues to adjust my program as needed. If you want to be the best you can be, by all means lose weight and exercise. That is a great start. But to really achieve the maximum benefits of modern science, you need the help of a first-rate and experienced longevity physician. The trick is to find a really great doctor you can work with who specializes in this field.

There are a lot of doctors out there doing longevity medicine. And, as in every field, most are competent, a few are miserable fakes, and a few at the other end of the spectrum are great healers. The trick is telling who is who. I can't give you much guidance in a book about who are the greats and who should be avoided at all costs. I know the skills of the doctors in my clinic because I work with them daily. I have a big hand in keeping them up to date on the rapid changes. So of course, I recommend them. But I am clearly biased!

If you are in the Seattle area, our clinics are located in:

KIRKLAND:
9757 Juanita Drive NE
Suite 200
Kirkland, WA 98034
Phone: 425-576-9272

TACOMA:
3315 S. 23rd Street
Suite 204
Tacoma, WA 98405
Phone: 253-682-4100

LYNNWOOD:
19221 36th Avenue W
Suite 210
Lynnwood, WA 98036
Phone: 425-670-1000

For more information, go to our website at longevitymedicalclinic.com.
You can read about and buy our supplements at:
longevitymedicalclinic.com.

Notes

Introduction

A dramatic fall in life expectancy
https://www.health.harvard.edu/blog/why-life-expectancy-in-the-us-is-falling-202210202835#:~:text=With%20rare%20exceptions%2C%20life%20expectancy,risen%20to%20nearly%2079%20years

Overweight & Obesity Statistics
https://www.niddk.nih.gov/health-information/health-statistics/overweight-obesity

Diabetes and its drivers: the largest epidemic in human history
https://clindiabetesendo.biomedcentral.com/articles/10.1186/s40842-016-0039-3

Number of Americans with diabetes to double or triple by 2050
https://www.cdc.gov/media/pressrel/2010/r101022.html

Diabetes Complications
https://www.ncbi.nlm.nih.gov/pmc/articles/PMC3870323/

Epidemiology of Diabetes and Diabetes-Related
https://www.endocrine.org/patient-engagement/endocrine-library/diabetes-complications

Chapter 1

Muscle tissue changes with aging
https://www.ncbi.nlm.nih.gov/pmc/articles/PMC2804956/

Female Age-Related Fertility Decline
https://www.acog.org/clinical/clinical-guidance/committee-opinion/articles/2014/03/female-age-related-fertility-decline

Hair Loss in Women
https://my.clevelandclinic.org/health/diseases/16921-hair-loss-in-women

Erectile Dysfunction
https://www.clevelandclinicmeded.com/medicalpubs/diseasemanagement/endocrinology/erectile-dysfunction/

Loss of Libido
https://www.ncbi.nlm.nih.gov/pmc/articles/PMC5722087/

Diets Do Not Work
https://slate.com/technology/2015/03/diets-do-not-work-the-thin-evidence-that-losing-weight-makes-you-healthier.html

Chapter 2

Adult Obesity Facts
https://www.cdc.gov/obesity/data/adult.html

Breast Cancer and hormone therapy. The Women's Health Initiative Hormone Therapy Trials
https://www.ncbi.nlm.nih.gov/pmc/articles/PMC3963523/

Testosterone and Breast Cancer Prevention
https://pubmed.ncbi.nlm.nih.gov/26160683/

Breast Cancer Incidence Reduction in Women Treated with Subcutaneous Testosterone https://pubmed.ncbi.nlm.nih.gov/33870115/

Testosterone therapy in breast cancer survivors
https://www.researchgate.net/publication/360529284_Glaser_AS_TT_in_BCA_survivors

Breast Cancer Incidence Reduction in Women Treated with Subcutaneous Testosterone: https://www.ncbi.nlm.nih.gov/pmc/articles/PMC8025725/

Progesterone suppresses the invasion and migration of breast cancer cells
https://www.ncbi.nlm.nih.gov/pmc/articles/PMC5537311/

Progesterone vs. synthetic progestins and the risk of breast cancer
https://pubmed.ncbi.nlm.nih.gov/27456847/

Cognitive function and the benefits of pregnenolone supplements
https://supplementengineer.com/blogs/supplements/pregnenolone

GH (growth hormone) and the cardiovascular system: an update on a topic at heart
https://link.springer.com/article/10.1007/s12020-014-0327-6

Age-dependent impairment of endothelial progenitor cells is corrected by growth-hormone-mediated increase of insulin-like growth-factor -1https://pubmed.ncbi.nlm.nih.gov/17234973/
Could transdermal estradiol + progesterone be a safer postmenopausal HRT? A review
https://www.sciencedirect.com/science/article/abs/pii/S0378512208002041

HRT optimization, using transdermal estradiol plus micronized progesterone, a safer HRT
https://pubmed.ncbi.nlm.nih.gov/18775609/

Chapter 3

The 2020-2025 Dietary Guidelines for Americans
https://medlineplus.gov/ency/patientinstructions/000838.htm

By Age Fifty, the Average Woman has Lost 50% of her Estrogens
https://www.straighthealthcare.com/female-hormone-physiology.html

Relationship between low levels of anabolic hormones and 6-year mortality in older men
https://pubmed.ncbi.nlm.nih.gov/17998499/

Two Former New England Compounding Center Pharmacists Sentenced
https://www.justice.gov/usao-ma/pr/two-former-new-england-compounding-center-pharmacists-sentenced

Number of Americans with diabetes to double or triple by 2050
https://www.cdc.gov/media/pressrel/2010/r101022.html

The Disease Burden Associated with Overweight and Obesity
https://jamanetwork.com/journals/jama/fullarticle/192030

Obesity and Its Related Diseases: A New Escalating Alarming in Global Health
https://www.paradigmpress.org/jimr/article/view/505

Obesity increases the risk for severe COVID-19–associated illness
https://www.cdc.gov/mmwr/volumes/70/wr/mm7010e4.htm

Body Mass Index and Risk for COVID-19–Related Hospitalization, Intensive Care Unit Admission, Invasive Mechanical Ventilation, and Death
https://www.cdc.gov/mmwr/volumes/70/wr/mm7010e4.htm

Effect of the COVID-19 pandemic on obesity and its risk factors
https://link.springer.com/article/10.1186/s12889-023-15833-2

20 Things you Didn't Know About the Human gut Microbiome
https://www.ncbi.nlm.nih.gov/pmc/articles/PMC4191858/

Postbiotics
https://www.ncbi.nlm.nih.gov/pmc/articles/PMC9027423/

From degenerative disease to malignant tumors: Insight to the function of ApoE
https://www.sciencedirect.com/science/article/pii/S0753332222015165

APOE4 is associated with cognitive and pathological heterogeneity in patients with Alzheimer's disease: a systematic review
https://alzres.biomedcentral.com/articles/10.1186/s13195-020-00712-4

Life style habits associated with lower Alzheimer disease risk
https://www.ncbi.nlm.nih.gov/pmc/articles/PMC3207358/

Impacts of microplastics on immunity
https://www.ncbi.nlm.nih.gov/pmc/articles/PMC9552327/

Senolytics in idiopathic pulmonary fibrosis: Results from a first-in-human, open-label, pilot study
https://pubmed.ncbi.nlm.nih.gov/30616998/

Use of sirolimus in solid organ transplantation
https://pubmed.ncbi.nlm.nih.gov/17335296/

Chapter 4

Nutrition as We Age: Healthy Eating with the Dietary Guidelines https://health.gov/news/202107/nutrition-we-age-healthy-eating-dietary-guidelines

Understanding the Value of the Wellness Visit
https://www.ncbi.nlm.nih.gov/pmc/articles/PMC8455445/

Surprising dangers of vitamins and supplements
https://www.consumerreports.org/cro/magazine/2012/09/10-surprising-dangers-of-vitamins-and-supplements/index.htm

Chapter 5

Overdose deaths from prescription drugs
https://nida.nih.gov/research-topics/trends-statistics/overdose-death-rates#:~:text=Drug%20overdose%20deaths%20involving%20prescription,involving%20prescription%20opioids%20totaled%2016%2C706

Brand and generic medications: Are they interchangeable?
https://www.ncbi.nlm.nih.gov/pmc/articles/PMC6074234/

Report details where top 100 brand-name Rx drugs are made
https://www.cidrap.umn.edu/report-details-where-top-100-brand-name-rx-drugs-are-made

Vitamin D Deficiency, Osteoporosis and Effect on Autoimmune Diseases and Hematopoiesis: A Review
https://www.ncbi.nlm.nih.gov/pmc/articles/PMC8396272/

Role of Vitamin D
https://www.emerald.com/insight/content/doi/10.1108/AGJSR-04-2022-0028/full/html

Role of Vitamin D
https://publications.aap.org/pediatrics/article-abstract/129/3/485/31795/Maternal-Serum-Vitamin-D-Levels-During-Pregnancy?redirectedFrom=fulltext

Effect of Vitamin D3 Supplementation in the First 2 Years of Life on Psychiatric Symptoms at Ages 6 to 8 Years
https://jamanetwork.com/journals/jamanetworkopen/fullarticle/2805032

Curcumin Synergizes With Resveratrol to Inhibit Colon Cancer
https://www.ncbi.nlm.nih.gov/pmc/articles/PMC6370344/#:~:text=Curcumin%20together%20with%20resveratrol%20causes,regimen%20of%20curcumin%20and%20resveratrol.

Dehydroepiandrosterone (DHEA)
https://www.mountsinai.org/health-library/supplement/dehydroepiandrosterone

Comprehensive Review on Phytochemicals, Pharmacological and Clinical Potentials of Gymnema sylvestre
https://www.ncbi.nlm.nih.gov/pmc/articles/PMC6830388/

Building strength, endurance, and mobility using an astaxanthin formulation
https://pubmed.ncbi.nlm.nih.gov/30259703/

Astaxanthin, cell membrane nutrient with diverse clinical benefits and anti-aging potential
https://pubmed.ncbi.nlm.nih.gov/22214255/

Chapter 6

Benefits of Physical Activity
https://www.cdc.gov/physicalactivity/basics/pa-health/index.htm#:~:text=Regular%20physical%20activity%20is%20one,ability%20to%20do%20everyday%20activities

Physical activity with mortality reduction among breast cancer survivors.
https://www.medicalnewstoday.com/articles/15-minutes-of-physical-activity-may-reduce-breast-cancer-mortality-by-60#:~:text=%E2%80%9CThe%20study%20found%20that%20even,were%20more%20active%2C%E2%80%9D%20Dr

For Women with Breast Cancer, Regular Exercise May Improve Survival
https://www.cancer.gov/news-events/cancer-currents-blog/2020/breast-cancer-survival-exercise

7,000 steps a day reduced middle-aged people's risk of premature death.
https://sph.unc.edu/sph-news/how-many-steps-lead-to-longevity-study-identifies-new-daily-goals/#:~:text=The%20new%20research%20supports%20and,people%27s%20risk%20of%20premature%20death.

Chapter 7

Arthritis Fact Sheet
https://www.cdc.gov/chronicdisease/resources/publications/factsheets/arthritis.htm

Inflammation plays a key role in osteoarthritis, just as it does in most other types of arthritis
https://www.ncbi.nlm.nih.gov/pmc/articles/PMC4870316

Hip fracture as risk factor for mortality in patients over 65 years of age
https://pubmed.ncbi.nlm.nih.gov/26016287/#:~:text=Abstract,process%20and%20its%20dire%20consequences

Femoral neck fracture is a common injury in the elderly, and its incidence is rising in parallel with an increase in traffic accidents and population aging
https://www.ncbi.nlm.nih.gov/pmc/articles/PMC4870316/

A BMI less than 18.5 means you're underweight; 18.5 to 24.9 is a healthy weight range; 25.0 to 29.9 is overweight; and 30.0 or higher is obese
https://www.nhlbi.nih.gov/health/educational/lose_wt/index.htm

Reducing Calorie Intake May Not Help You Lose Body Weight
https://www.ncbi.nlm.nih.gov/pmc/articles/PMC5639963/

Exercise facilitates weight control, partly through effects on appetite regulation.
https://pubmed.ncbi.nlm.nih.gov/30131457/

Acute and Chronic Effects of Exercise on Appetite, Energy Intake, and Appetite-Related Hormones
https://pubmed.ncbi.nlm.nih.gov/30131457/

Chapter 8

Influence of intermittent fasting on human health
https://www.ncbi.nlm.nih.gov/pmc/articles/PMC4516560/

Impact of intermittent fasting on health and disease processes https://pubmed.ncbi.nlm.nih.gov/27810402/

The Effect of Fasting on Human Metabolism and Psychological Health
https://pubmed.ncbi.nlm.nih.gov/35035610/

Fiber and the effect of the gut microbiome on weight regulation
https://www.nature.com/articles/s41467-023-38778-x

The potential effects from long-term use of non-sugar sweeteners such as an increased risk of type 2 diabetes, cardiovascular diseases, and mortality in adults
https://www.who.int/news/item/15-05-2023-who-advises-not-to
-use-non-sugar-sweeteners-for-weight-control-in-newly-released
-guideline#:~:text=%C2%A9-,WHO%20advises%20not%20to%20
use%20non%2Dsugar%20sweeteners%20for,control%20in%20
newly%20released%20guideline&text=The%20World%20Health%20
Organization%20(WHO,of%20noncommunicable%20diseases%20
(NCDs)

Caffeine: How much is too much
https://www.mayoclinic.org/healthy-lifestyle/nutrition-and-healthy
-eating/in-depth/caffeine/art-20045678

Green tea and weight loss
https://www.healthline.com/nutrition/green-tea-and-weight-loss

Sildenafil inhibits the growth of human colorectal cancer in vitro and in vivo
https://pubmed.ncbi.nlm.nih.gov/26807313/

Tadalafil augments tumor specific immunity in patients with head and neck squamous cell carcinoma
https://pubmed.ncbi.nlm.nih.gov/30510089/

Chapter 9

Inflammation and dementia
https://www.ncbi.nlm.nih.gov/pmc/articles/PMC3390758/

Erectile dysfunction drugs increase brain flow and improve cognition
https://www.ncbi.nlm.nih.gov/pmc/articles/PMC6705107/

Structural brain changes in aging: courses, causes and cognitive consequences
https://pubmed.ncbi.nlm.nih.gov/20879692/

Brain size, sex, and the aging brain
https://pubmed.ncbi.nlm.nih.gov/25161056/

The Role of Estrogen in Brain and Cognitive Aging
https://pubmed.ncbi.nlm.nih.gov/31364065/

Emotional and cognitive functional imaging of estrogen and progesterone effects in the female human brain: a systematic review
https://pubmed.ncbi.nlm.nih.gov/25222701/

Estrogen, brain structure, and cognition in postmenopausal women
https://pubmed.ncbi.nlm.nih.gov/32910516/

Long-term effects of resveratrol on cognition, cerebrovascular function and cardio-metabolic markers in postmenopausal women: A 24-month randomized, double-blind, placebo-controlled, crossover study
https://pubmed.ncbi.nlm.nih.gov/32900519/

Resveratrol Boosts Cognitive Function by Targeting SIRT1 https://pubmed.ncbi.nlm.nih.gov/29943083/
Effects of creatine supplementation on cognitive function of healthy individuals: A systematic review of randomized controlled trials
https://www.ncbi.nlm.nih.gov/pmc/articles/PMC6093191/

Nutritional Supplements and the Brain
https://www.frontiersin.org/articles/10.3389/fnagi.2019.00056/full

Roles of taurine in cognitive function of physiology, pathologies and toxication
https://pubmed.ncbi.nlm.nih.gov/31220527/

Chapter 10

Oxytocin vaginal gel could significantly improve vaginal atrophy and sexual function in postmenopausal women
https://pubmed.ncbi.nlm.nih.gov/32169019/

Improving vaginal health
https://academic.oup.com/smr/article-abstract/8/3/379/6880238

Associations between Dopamine D4 Receptor Gene Variation with Both Infidelity and Sexual Promiscuity
https://www.researchgate.net/publication/49678095_Associations_between_Dopamine_D4_Receptor_Gene_Variation_with_Both_Infidelity_and_Sexual_Promiscuity

Incidence rate of prostate cancer in men treated for erectile dysfunction with phosphodiesterase type 5 inhibitors: retrospective analysis
https://pubmed.ncbi.nlm.nih.gov/23353723/

Chapter 11

Life's biggest stressors
https://www.stress.org/holmes-rahe-stress-inventory

Skin cancer rates are skyrocketing
https://www.skincancer.org/skin-cancer-information/skin-cancer-facts/

Netherlands will dish out free sun cream to residents in bid to tackle soaring skin cancer rates
https://www.dailymail.co.uk/health/article-12189459/Netherlands-dish-free-sun-cream-residents-bid-tackle-soaring-skin-cancer-rates.html

Chapter 12

Sleep deprivation can cause serious health issues
https://www.medicalnewstoday.com/articles/324799

The use and misuse of melatonin in the treatment of sleep disorders
https://pubmed.ncbi.nlm.nih.gov/30148726/

Index

E

H

M

N

O

P

T

Made in United States
Troutdale, OR
05/08/2024